Boys to Men in the Shadow of AIDS

Boys to Men in the Shadow of AIDS

Masculinities and HIV Risk in Zambia

Anthony Simpson

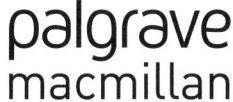

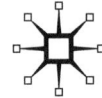

BOYS TO MEN IN THE SHADOW OF AIDS
Copyright © Anthony Simpson, 2009.

All rights reserved.

Portions of this work have been previously published.

Chapter 2 is a revised version of "Sons and Fathers/Boys to Men in the Time of AIDS: Learning Masculinity in Zambia." *Journal of Southern African Studies* 31 (3): 569–586. Taylor and Francis. 2005.

Chapter 3 is an expanded version of "Learning Sex and Gender in Zambia: Masculinities and HIV/AIDS Risk." *Sexualities* 10 (2): 173–188. Sage Publications. 2007.

Some extracts are taken from "Courage, Conquest and Condoms." In *"AIDS, Culture and Africa,"* ed. Douglas A. Feldman. University of Florida Press. 2008.

Permission to publish this material here is gratefully acknowledged.

First published in 2009 by
PALGRAVE MACMILLAN®
in the United States—a division of St. Martin's Press LLC,
175 Fifth Avenue, New York, NY 10010.

Where this book is distributed in the UK, Europe and the rest of the world, this is by Palgrave Macmillan, a division of Macmillan Publishers Limited, registered in England, company number 785998, of Houndmills, Basingstoke, Hampshire RG21 6XS.

Palgrave Macmillan is the global academic imprint of the above companies and has companies and representatives throughout the world.

Palgrave® and Macmillan® are registered trademarks in the United States, the United Kingdom, Europe and other countries.

ISBN-13: 978-0-230-61391-1
ISBN-10: 0-230-61391-8

Library of Congress Cataloging-in-Publication Data is available from the Library of Congress.

A catalogue record of the book is available from the British Library.

Design by Newgen Imaging Systems (P) Ltd., Chennai, India.

First edition: May 2009

10 9 8 7 6 5 4 3 2 1

Printed in the United States of America.

Contents

Acknowledgments	vii
1. Introduction	1
2. Fathers and Sons: The Measure of a Man	19
3. Learning Sex In and Out of School	37
4. Sexual Lives after School	61
5. Married Life	91
6. Sexuality as a Site of Difference	115
7. "Has God Come in Another Way?"	145
8. Responses to Campaigns	171
9. Conclusion	193
Notes	205
References	221
Index	235

Acknowledgments

Many people have assisted me in the long process of writing this book. I am grateful to Ronnie Frankenberg for his encouragement at the outset of the project. Friends and colleagues read my work as it progressed. Some commented on the whole manuscript, while others read chapters of earlier versions. I am grateful to Elizabeth Colson, Jeanette Edwards, Gillian Evans, Harri Englund, James Ferguson, Suzette Heald, Paul Henley, David Mills, Robert Morrell, Judith Okely, Lyn Schumaker, Tom Yarrow, and Soumhya Venkatesan for their helpful comments and advice. I would also like to thank heads of the department of Social Anthropology at Manchester University, John Gledhill at the project's inception, and Sarah Green at its conclusion for their help and encouragement. I am also indebted to Austin Cheyeka in Zambia and to my nephew Paul in England, and to Marie Rostron and Lynn Dignan at Manchester University for their generous practical assistance. Luba Ostashevsky, Colleen Lawrie, and Allison McElgunn at Palgrave have shepherded the book through its various stages with kindness and expertise. Maran Elancheran has provided excellent copyediting.

Members of my family, my mother Lois, my sisters Susan, Maureen, and Catherine and their partners George, Bill, and Alex have given constant encouragement and support. Most of all I am indebted to the Zambian men and women who agreed to take part in this research. They allowed me access to some of the intimate spaces of their lives. They trusted that I would use the information I learned in a responsible manner. I have tried my best to honor that trust.

1

INTRODUCTION

Sampa and Promise, Paul and Kangwa, Darius, Henry, and their classmates were students together at a Zambian boys' Catholic mission boarding school in the early 1980s. These are not their real names. I have used pseudonyms and at times altered superficial details about them to protect their anonymity in this account of their lives, lived in the shadow of HIV/AIDS. My research focuses on a number of questions; among them: How did they learn to be men? How did they come to know themselves as engendered sexual beings? How have they conducted their sexual lives in the face of the pandemic?

I taught these men in the junior and senior secondary stages of their education, at the school that I call St. Antony's, where I was a teacher through much of the 1970s, 1980s, and the early and mid 1990s. They belonged to the "fortunate few" Zambians "lucky" enough to win places at one of the best schools in the country. They formed part of an elite in terms of educational opportunity, though this did not necessarily ensure elite membership twenty years later. They came from a wide range of socioeconomic backgrounds. Many were the children of subsistence farmers and manual laborers. Others came from wealthier households with fathers in professional work or in the higher echelons of the ruling political party, the United National Independence Party (UNIP). Several were the sons of primary school teachers. I watched them grow from shy newcomers in their early and mid-teens—*kwiyos* in student talk[1]—to confident school-leavers. Many were impatient to fulfil their dreams of what they imagined education would deliver—to become doctors, lawyers, engineers, teachers—and to achieve the status of adult men by marrying and having children. Some did indeed achieve their aims, though others faced lives of poverty and unemployment and some lives were cut short by AIDS.

When I first recorded their life histories in 1983 and 1984, around the time they finished school, my interest was to explore the impact of Catholic mission education. They were then mainly in their late teens or early twenties.[2] Interviews covered a wide range of topics. Students recalled their childhood; they spoke about their religious beliefs and their hopes and fears for the future. They candidly described their childhood and adolescent sexual activity. In our early conversations the topic of HIV/AIDS did not figure. It was not yet on their horizon.

However, in 1983, less than 100 miles away at the University Teaching Hospital in Zambia's capital, Lusaka, Dr. Anne Bayley, professor of surgery, was confronted with an unusual number of patients suffering from aggressive Kaposi's sarcoma (a type of cancer) and who did not respond to routine therapy (Bayley 1984; Bayley et al. 1985; Bayley 1996). When these patients were tested in 1984, 91 percent of them proved to be HIV-positive. Bayley later concluded that HIV had probably arrived in Zambia in the mid-1970s.[3] During the 1980s, news of AIDS slowly began to filter through to young Zambians. Early designations of AIDS as a "gay plague" persuaded former students of St. Antony's, like many young men throughout Zambia, to conclude that AIDS posed no threat to them. "It's you Europeans who are all homosexuals," they regularly assured me. "We Africans, we like our women!" When they came to understand that AIDS in Africa was spread predominantly through heterosexual sex, many young men were convinced that they could tell simply by looking whether a girl had the HIV virus. In the face of my repeated protests that it was not possible to identify those who were HIV-positive by looking at them, successive cohorts of students said they understood that it took "a long time" to die from AIDS, and that death in another form might well find them before they succumbed to the disease. As campaigns went on to target "risk groups"—prostitutes and long-distance truck drivers—none of us anticipated the way in which AIDS would come to dominate everyday life in Zambia.[4]

Zambia (formerly Northern Rhodesia) is one of the countries most severely affected by HIV/AIDS in the sub-Saharan region where the pandemic has taken the most terrible toll to date, with 2 percent of the world's population and by 2004 nearly 30 percent of its HIV cases (Iliffe 2006: 33). The 2007 UNAIDS epidemic update notes that, while there is little sign of decline in the HIV prevalence of 17 percent at the national level in Zambia, there was some decline in some parts of the country (UNAIDS 2007: 17).[5] Between 1994 and 2004 the overall HIV prevalence remained relatively stable at 19–20 percent among pregnant women aged fifteen to thirty-nine years (UNAIDS Update 2006). The 2006 update further observed, "At current levels of HIV prevalence, young persons in Zambia face a 50% life-time risk of dying of AIDS, in the absence of treatment (Ministry of Health Zambia 2005)." Of almost 1 million adults (15–49) and children (0–14 years) in Zambia estimated to be living with HIV in 2003 (UNICEF 2006), over 85,000 were children, while an estimated 1.1 million children (0–18) had been orphaned, mostly due to HIV/AIDS (UNICEF 2007). The early spread and impact of the pandemic was exacerbated by Zambia's economic decline, increasing indebtedness, and World Bank programs that caused health services to introduce user fees that resulted in an 80 percent drop in utilization of urban health centers.[6] Parker notes that the same World Bank later became the main funder of HIV/AIDS prevention work in the developing world, "leading the global fight against an epidemic that its own previous policies did much to structure" (Parker 2000: 44).

I had initially interviewed a cohort of twenty-four students in 1983 and 1984. I reinterviewed twelve of the survivors of the original cohort almost twenty years later in 2002. I again collected life histories and discussed their sexual activity. Few men were in regular contact with any of their former classmates though they might know where some of them were living and what occupations they had. Still, they remained proud of their shared identity as "old boys" of St. Antony's. One former student, Demba, declined to be reinterviewed. Though happy to meet socially, he explained that he felt his life had been so unhappy that he had no desire to recall, and, in a sense, to "relive" it. By 2002, eight of the original group had died, as had five of their wives, most of them, their friends and relatives assumed, from AIDS-related conditions. I was unable to locate the other three. I contacted a further eighteen former students, school contemporaries of the original cohort. They were interviewed, as were twelve former students' wives, one widow, and other male and female household members.[7] During twelve months' ethnographic fieldwork I lived in the homes of some of the former students and participated in their everyday lives. My account is informed by this experience, as I draw upon my observations and on the many casual conversations that contributed to our shared sociality. I had further contact with many of the men and their families during brief research trips to Zambia each year from 2004 to 2007.

In 2002 the age range of the former students in this study was between thirty-five and the early forties. They belonged to a number of ethnic groups, primarily Bemba and Tonga, but also included Lala, Ila, Chikunda, Lamba, and Lozi.[8] Though very few men, unlike their wives, regularly attended church, all claimed a Christian identity, as they had done at secondary school, the majority of them Catholic—though religious affiliations also included Seventh Day Adventist, United Church of Zambia, Jehovah's Witnesses, Assemblies of God, and various Pentecostal churches. About 25 percent of the Zambian population is estimated to be Catholic in this predominantly Christian country. The Catholic Church in Zambia has played, and continues to play, a significant role in the provision of secondary education as it does in the care of those suffering from AIDS and in its opposition to condoms as a method of HIV prevention. There was a wide range of income within the group of former students, some men earning as much as 7 million kwacha (about U.S. $1,550) a month and some as little as 100, 000 kwacha (about U.S. $22) a month or less.[9] Occupations included the following: doctors, lawyers, managers, lecturers, teachers, engineers, petrol pump attendants, security guards, and "businessmen"—the latter generally were involved in informal trading. Several respondents were unemployed. All thirty were resident in urban areas or provincial centers. All except two were married, and many of the marriages were interethnic. Some wives were in professional employment; some were marketers and traders. Others were housewives with no employment beyond the household.

Several former students I contacted were in poor health. While men often portrayed themselves as "survivors"—of Zambia's severe economic decline and of the decimation of their generation by AIDS—the pandemic threw its shadow over many of our encounters. All the men in this study had lost family members, friends, and work colleagues to AIDS. Many of them suspected that they were HIV-positive. At times, grief and depression threatened to overwhelm them. Several had been entrusted with the support of their siblings' orphaned children. All the men had the information and the means at their disposal to protect themselves and their sexual partners from the risk of exposure to the HIV virus. This ethnography is about why, in striving to appear "real" men, many at times chose not to do so.

I conducted fieldwork among a small group of men who coincidentally happened to be drawn to St. Antony's during the time I was teaching there. I was able to establish sufficient rapport for them to share with me intimate details of their lives both in youth and adulthood. Anthropologists have often chosen to work on a "small" scale in order to gain in-depth understandings of the complex lives of others by detailed qualitative exploration of the contexts of such lives and by revealing the meanings people attach to their embodied experience. Ethnographies can provide "textured firsthand accounts" (Schoepf 1992: 260) that may lead to vital insights inaccessible to other approaches and, indeed, complement them. They may reveal patterns of social behavior while at the same time record exceptions to such patterns, thereby avoiding unwarranted generalizations. (See Cohen 1996.) The tragedy of HIV/AIDS calls for flexible multidisciplinary approaches. An anthropological monograph offers very specific knowledge, but knowledge, as Okely (1996) observes, "with which others can engage." While revealing diversity in their responses to the possibilities open to them to perform their manliness, former students throw light upon aspects of sexual life that many men share. In this ethnography I draw attention to, at times striking, similarities in other accounts of men's lives in Zambia, in Africa, and beyond.

Why Men and Masculinities Matter in the HIV/AIDS Pandemic

Early awareness of the uneven gendered impact of the pandemic led to a focus primarily on women's physiological, economic, social, and cultural vulnerability. Some responses to HIV/AIDS promoted the remedicalization of sexuality (Parker et al. 2000) and individualistic behavioral approaches. However, social anthropologists, among others, have insisted that attention be paid to global political economy and to the dynamics of gender power relations.[10] Global forces necessarily play an important role in the construction of masculine identities and the local can only be understood within larger global frames. Such large-scale forces as colonialism and its aftermath (Stoler 1991), religion, the state, mass media, and markets (Connell 2000: 89) shape sex. In Zambia, imperialism and global capitalism have had a significant impact on gender identities. Ethnographers of Zambian marriage and families have long documented shifts among matrilineal groups, such as Bemba and Tonga, in the balance of roles between father and mother's brother, and between husband and wife.

My focus on men is not to deny the importance of studies that have argued for the need to put women at the center of analysis. (See, for example, Reid 1997a.) Women bear the brunt of the multifaceted consequences of the AIDS pandemic. Men's sexuality has serious, often fatal, consequences for women. Many women are particularly at risk and in need of empowerment because of men's violence. Violence and the threat of violence, for example, increase women's inability to negotiate condom use. What is perhaps less self-evident in view of the real power exercised by many men in everyday life in Zambia and elsewhere is the vulnerability of men because of the demands made upon them by particular constructions of masculinity. Wilton and Aggleton have insisted, "It is the hegemonic status of masculinity, predicated upon the subordination of women, which presented the greatest challenge in our struggle against the epidemic" (1991: 156). However, care must be taken not to present some simplistic notion of gender and dominance. It is generally recognized that we should not expect to find one single gender ideology in any society but rather a number of apparently contradictory ones, all of them constructed, and shaped, by a myriad of social and historical forces, and negotiable in varying degrees. (See Connell 1995, 2000; Meigs 1990; Sanders 1999.)

Many commentators have emphasized the need for research into concepts of virility and masculinities, and into men's roles in the transmission of HIV (Ankrah 1991; de Bruyn 1992; Obbo 1993, 1995; Campbell 1995; Rivers and Aggleton 1999; Foreman 1999; Setel 1999; Bujra 2000; Baylies and Bujra with the Gender and AIDS Group 2000). A shift in focus by international agencies toward men and masculinities was signaled by organizations such as the Joint United Nations Program on HIV/AIDS (UNAIDS) dedicating its 2000–2001 World AIDS Campaign as "Men and AIDS: A Gendered Approach." Peter Piot, the head of the UNAIDS organization, argued: "Men are the key to reducing HIV transmission and have the power to change the course of the AIDS epidemic" (UNAIDS 2001). However, as Silberschmidt (2004), among others, has noted, such statements risked essentializing the category "men," screening from view the complexities of multiple masculinities. Plummer, in addition, points to the need to recognize multiple male sexualities and to acknowledge that "much sexual action will take different pathways from that of the hegemonic model" (2005: 187).

There is a continuing need to "bring men in" in efforts to combat the pandemic. Many have argued that masculinity is in need of reconstruction and of reshaping. Yet, how best to achieve this? The recognition that masculinities are historically, socially, and economically constructed, and that gender is a process, offers the potential for change. However, in Zambia as elsewhere in Africa, little is known about men's perceptions of themselves as engendered sexual beings. How do they arrive at these perceptions? What is the relationship between these and their sexual conduct in African contexts where, in Morrell and Swart's depiction, "compulsory heterosexuality is a key feature of hegemonic masculinity" (2005: 107). Zambian government demographic and health surveys are indicative, but fine-grained analyses of the ways in which men relate to constructions of masculinity, their beliefs and their projects, and the range of subject positions taken or assigned over the life cycle are missing. Despite such wildly optimistic comments as "[t]he only vaccine to combat HIV/AIDS is education" (UNESCO workshop proceedings 2001), it has become generally recognized that the communication of Western biomedical "knowledge" alone will not curtail the spread of HIV/AIDS. More needs to be learned about the contexts in which the transmission of HIV takes place and in which health messages are constructed, transmitted, and received (see Heald 2002). "Context" needs to be understood as a dynamic process, as Dowsett comments, to connote "the historical and institutional nature and organization of human interactions and meaning-making (i.e. this is context as actively constructive)" (1999: 98).

HIV/AIDS prevention messages may appear totally inappropriate when situated within other explanatory discourses. As Lupton has noted, in many campaigns sexuality is assumed to be contained within the individual who can exercise rational control in a straightforward manner. Yet, she observes: "The discourse on safer sex assumes that pleasure and desire can be reorganized in response to imperatives based on health risks.... However, the dominant way in which people understand sexuality is, perhaps, in terms of irrationality, passion and irresistibility" (Lupton 1995: 88).

I would also argue that people may conduct their sexual lives in accordance with a different logic of sexual practice, a different logic of desire from that which informs health campaigns. This ethnography demonstrates the rational manner in which a group of Zambian men express and experience their sexuality. There are other risks at stake, apart from the risk to health. For many former students, the risk of failing to act as "real men" in their sexual lives dictated the choices they made in their performance of masculinity.

My aim in this book is to excavate the mainsprings of adult male identity formation among a group of Zambian men in an attempt to understand gender relations and their expression in sexual encounters in the midst of the pandemic. Using firsthand accounts, I explore the ways in which many men—like women—are vulnerable in the pandemic, endangered by ideologies of masculinity that lead them to ignore prevention messages and to engage in sex that makes them vulnerable to HIV infection. Parker has noted that if interventions are to succeed "they must respond to the nuances of cultural particularity and detail" (1992: 240). He suggests that it is possible to approach the erotic much as we would examine a system of religious beliefs, or a particular political ideology, and encourages researchers to go beyond the empirical frequency of certain sexual acts in order to comprehend "the emotional power that they hold for the participants and the wider systems of meaning that make them significant" (ibid.: 226). This requires nuanced qualitative accounts of sexual experience.

There is no pretence here that the men form an undifferentiated category free of contestation. In Zambia, as elsewhere (Connell 1995: 54), hegemonic forms of masculinity remain subject to challenge. Heald points to the way in which ideas of masculinity, under the influence of feminism, "are now seen as fractured into a diversity of images and lived out in a multitude of ways" (1999: 2). However, in his recent study of the lives of nine Ghanaian men, *Making Men in Ghana*, Miescher rejects postcolonial characterizations of a fragmented or fractured self, commenting: "[I]n narrating their selves, the men at the center of this study created selves and acted as subjects that in their view were not problematic, fragmented, or in need of liberation" (2005: 15). At least some of the Zambian men in my study recognize that alleviation of the devastating consequences of the HIV/AIDS pandemic will entail the liberation of both men and women from prevailing gender regimes.

I have no intention to demonize men. Nothing is to be gained by presenting my informants as either heroes or antiheroes (see Caplan 1997: 229). Nor is it my objective to essentialize either men or women, each variously situated in constantly shifting fields of power, and thereby to elide differences among them. (See Uebel 1997: 5.) However, a clear profile emerges from former students' accounts, irrespective of ethnic identity or religious affiliation, about prevailing ideologies concerning what it meant for them to be men, "real men," and hence how they constituted relationships—both with women and with other men. The efforts a group of Zambian men made either to "live up to" expectations of manliness in their sexual lives, to forego or resist such efforts, are documented here. At the core of the prevailing hegemonic version of masculinity was the demonstration of male potency in sexual conquest. While there *were* exceptions, throughout childhood and adolescence (as indeed in adulthood) sexuality for many men was a space to create and restore masculinity. It was a sexuality that for almost all stressed technique and performance and that had as its focus penetration and speed of ejaculation.

My research reveals that many former students' sense of their manhood is something that has constantly to be achieved and reclaimed in the performance of masculinity in public- and in intimate spheres. Indeed in both spheres, masculinity may best be seen as a fragile entity, encompassed by a deep sense of insecurity most acutely felt within, and indeed particularly produced by, life within the male peer group. Reynaud has pointed to certain ironies in the embodiment of masculinity, commenting, "Man's misfortune is that his penis, the symbol of power, is in fact one of the most fragile and vulnerable organs of his body" (1981: 36). Kaufman (1998) highlights the complex fragility of masculinity:

> Masculinity is power. But masculinity is terrifyingly fragile because it does not really exist in the sense we are led to believe it exists, that is as a biological reality—something real that we have inside ourselves. It exists as ideology; it exists as scripted behavior; it exists within "gendered" relationships.... Yet boys and men harbor great insecurity about their male credentials. This insecurity exists because maleness is equated with masculinity. (1998: 8)

Several commentators have identified sexual performance as a crucial arena in which masculinity is socially constructed and enacted. (See, for example, Kimmel 1988.) Silberschmidt (2005: 197) notes how Kimmel's observation links up with Connell's (1995) contention that the essence of manhood is characterized in terms that to be a man is natural, healthy, and innate and contradictorily that a man must stay masculine and never let his masculinity falter. Tuzin has defined masculinity as "a thing of ideology and ontology" (1997: 181). Holland et al. (1998) have described how sexual risk-taking and sexual safety among young men and women in Britain are constituted in social relations of heterosexuality. Connell notes, "Masculinities do not exist prior to social interaction, but come into existence as people act" (2000: 218). And yet, as Weeks has observed, "the sexual is so much a mobile, changeable, culturally sensitive part of us and our culture, it is difficult to pin down" (1995: 12). Weeks highlights the enabling power of identities, but, like Butler (1990) and Hall (1996), he reminds us that identities are only ever provisional (Weeks 1995: 38).

I have chosen to investigate what for adult Zambians are considered to be "the secrets of the house," to seek to understand matters that have been described by one peer educator in Zambia as "too bedroom to know" (Kalipenta and Chalowandya 1995). The gap between representation and responsibility has been portrayed as the "master moral dilemma" (Kleinman et al. 1997: xii). If all representation risks the accusation of being pornography (Kappeler 1986), then investigations such as mine that focus mainly on sexual histories, how men think about sex and the kind of sex they engage in, run a particular risk. My research may appear particularly intrusive and prurient. It has been asserted that European culture has privileged sexuality as the essence of the self, a privileged "regime of truth" (Foucault 1979). Chapman and Rutherford (1988: 106) argue that the prevailing Western concept of sexuality already contains racism. As Fanon observed, "For the majority of white men the Negro represents the sexual instinct (in its raw state). The Negro is the incarnation of a genital potency beyond all moralities and prohibitions" (1967: 177). Because of the focus on black men's sexuality, I may stand accused of racism and voyeurism, exoticizing and hypersexualizing former students of St. Antony's, thereby perpetuating colonial and postcolonial fantasies of black men's sexuality (Chirimuuta and Chirimuuta 1987; Patton 1990; Setel 1999). Yet my intention is to shed light upon local knowledge about the meanings of manhood in Zambia, how these are expressed in sexual activity, and their role in the spread of HIV/AIDS. Central to this investigation is an exploration of power—the power men exercise over women, but also the power of ideologies of masculinity that imprison men. "Bringing men in" may well entail targeting them directly, and indeed confronting them about the hegemony of masculine definitions of sexual behavior (see Baylies and Bujra 2000: 179). This may risk anthropological research in AIDS prevention efforts becoming merely another form of social control (Clatts 1994; Thorogood 1992). However, anthropological research, sensitively conducted and disseminated, may contribute in enabling those most at risk and those dealing with the tragic consequences of the pandemic to discover the liberatory possibilities that AIDS brings in its wake.[11]

Life Histories

I have made extensive use of life histories—personal narrative material—in order to explore men's subjectivities, especially in relation to their sexual experience. I recognize, of course, that what are often missing in the accounts I collected are contests with others over memory. Because of the intimate nature of the material I was endeavoring to collect, these men produced their accounts for me in privacy and *as individuals*.[12] Marks reminds us that primary material like life stories presents the listener, or reader, "[n]ot so much with an historical world, but a certain consciousness of the world" (1989: 40). The study of sex presents particular methodological problems. Some commentators argue that the secondhand reports anthropologists have to rely on may well be filled with cultural idealization, myths, lies, denial, and underreporting (Herdt 1997: 11; Bolton 1992, 1995; Parker et al. 2000; Baylies and Bujra 2000: 51). Bolton observes that obtaining data on sexual encounters is "fraught with unreliability" (1992: 152). Green and Sobo note in the introduction to their joint study, "...we hope to avoid the easily-made mistake of equating what people say with what they do in practice" (2000: 12). Plummer also cautions the audience for such stories, "Whatever else a story is, it is not simply the lived life. It speaks all around the life.... But it is not *the* life, which is in principle unknown and unknowable" (1997: 168).

Caplan (1997: 230) points out that, in relating personal narratives, informants are required to grapple with their own self-identity. The data I present has been at least trebly mediated, first by my presence, then by the second-order reflection demanded from my informants, then by my later editing (see Rabinow 1977: 119). Former students and I have come to share something of a common history, thus making this research more than simply an intellectual exercise. However, in this instance, the ethnographer as audience is a former teacher to boot! I am aware of the caution required in attempting to analyze material, sometimes of a very intimate nature, recalled at my request, though what is considered intimate may vary between individuals and settings. My questions and their responses are indicative of the manner in which we reflected on one another and in which on each side of the encounter issues of self-presentation were salient.[13] During one of our interviews, before speaking about an extramarital affair, David broke off from his narrative to say, "And when I tell you this, I'm wondering, what are you going to think of me?"

Some men's accounts appear confessional in nature. They spoke of the relief they felt in having someone to discuss personal matters with, as they wrestled with how to conduct themselves, especially as husbands and fathers. As is only to be expected, the rapport between us differed from one man to the next, and from one meeting to another. At times interviewees presented me with a set of contradictions, as I doubtless did to them (see Mbilinyi 1989: 218). Nevertheless, my long-term continuing relationships with these men and the degree of trust built up over the years enabled me to discuss intimate aspects of male sexual conduct and to explore their sexual identities in some detail. I think that men's willingness to talk to me about their sexual experience was, at least in part, because we had been together throughout their secondary education. I had come to know some of them particularly well, partly because of the nature of boarding school life, and also because of my day-to-day interaction with them as clinic master and house master. And they had come to know me, their "mixed-race" teacher with a Trinidadian mother and an English father. Some students had expressed disappointment when they discovered that I was not really "white," but others were convinced that the African blood running through my veins helped me to understand them. Former students' readiness to speak frankly about their sexual activity was not complemented by a similar frankness from their wives who, in general, were less forthcoming in discussing sexual matters with my female local assistant. Evidently there was no shared history between them. Beyond this, notions of respectability restricted openness. Indicative of the unequal nature of some marriages, a few husbands refused wives permission to be interviewed. One wife independently declined to take part in the research.

Did some men feel coerced into speaking to me about the intimacies of their lives? When my research proposal was considered by the Manchester University ethics committee, the objection was raised that my informants might feel compelled to speak to me about their sexual lives because of our previous teacher-pupil relationship.[14] However, to several of the men interviewed I appeared to be someone who had not fulfilled his potential. I had "education," lots of it, but from the perspectives of lawyers, doctors, and others, I had signally failed to convert this learning into social and cultural capital. Former students' wives often commented upon my lack of achievement. Surveying the urban HIV/AIDS industry in Zambia, they told me that I should at least become a consultant and reap the rewards. Promise, like other former students, assured me that he did not feel compelled to speak with me. Yet one of our 2002 interviews in which we had discussed his recent extramarital sexual activity and the death of his brother from what he assumed was AIDS ended in this way:

TONY: Perhaps we can stop for today. I hope we haven't talked about anything that was too painful for you.
PROMISE: No, no. We haven't. I appreciate talking to you. I have to tell you the truth. There is nothing wrong.
TONY: Why do you say you have to tell me the truth?
PROMISE: Ah, whether I hide, or lie, or tell you the truth, well, it will still be the same. It's there. If it's there, so I have to say the truth! (Laughing.) Yes!

Almost all the interviews of former students were conducted in English. This was the language the men preferred. They said they felt they could express themselves better in English. Besides, in conversations with me, they found it easier to speak of sexual activity in a foreign language than in their first, Zambian language. They explained they would have found it embarrassing to speak about sexual matters in their own language to someone they perceived to be of their parents' generation. Vernacular appeared inappropriate, "too close." A few interviews, particularly with some of the men's parents and some of their wives, were conducted in Bemba, Tonga, or Nyanja. During all interviews, taped with the interviewees' permission, only the interviewer and interviewee were present. Some interviews were conducted in homes, others at places of work or recreation. Anonymity was assured at all times.

OUTLINE OF THE BOOK

Chapter 2 focuses on childhood and adolescence within the household. I highlight the father-son relationship, a relationship that most men characterized as one of fear. I do not intend to suggest that childhood experiences entirely determined later masculine identities. However, the father's example was always in the boy's eyes, even when a son might question his conduct. I explore the role of the father, as recalled by the men, in order to consider its significance for the particular nuances of masculine identity formation. Boys witnessed often-troubled relationships between their parents. Violent male discipline at home taught the adolescent the importance of toughness, of hiding fear and pain in the presence of others. This discipline did little to foster communication and the development of relationships of trust and care.[15] For many men this would have profound consequences, particularly in their relationships with wives and other sexual partners; when they suspected that they might be HIV-positive, they were unable to share their fears. The relationship with the mother, who often acted as a buffer between a boy and his father, was a notable exception. He was sure that she would *always* care for him, whatever the circumstances. This closeness between mother and son would endure. However, while husbands would readily reiterate the proverb, "Your wife is your mother," few of the men appeared able to establish such a relationship of trust with their wives or with other women who became their sexual partners.

In chapter 3 I outline the early sexual experiences of the cohort and highlight the crucial role of the peer group in developing constructions of masculinity. The chapter reveals adolescent anxieties and foreshadows their enduring significance in the men's adult lives. Men, unlike their wives and other female partners, readily described their first "adult" sexual experience—by "adult" they meant penetrative vaginal intercourse, when they first ejaculated into a girl. At times young men used force to achieve their aims. Men explained that, as adolescents, they understood coitus should be achieved with force and used violent imagery to describe this. In adolescence, as in adult life, many men spoke of the necessity of "firing several rounds" into a woman. They explained that they would often forego using condoms because of their need to prove their virility by the "strength" of their performance. The spoken and unspoken lessons of childhood and adolescence recalled by these Zambian men—and partially witnessed by me during their teenage years—provoked for many a restless anxiety to conform to an ideology of hegemonic masculinity. Among the consequences was sexual activity that put both men and women at risk in the HIV/AIDS pandemic.

Chapter 4 records the men's sexual activity after their schooldays and before they married. While about half of the original cohort went on to university in their pursuit of careers in law, medicine, and other professions, others sought various ways of making a living. Opportunities for further premarital sex are described. Many former students recalled feeling peer pressure to be known as sexually active. For all men, the ideal age for marriage was thirty. While most men married around this age, many explained it was their fear of AIDS that prompted them to wed. Men reasoned that marriage would protect them from AIDS, as they would be less likely to engage in unprotected sex with multiple partners if they had "sex" readily available at home. I sketch the circumstances around some of their marriages, their choice of partners, and highlight the importance of children. These "modern," "educated" men still adhered to the "tradition" of paying *lobola* (bridewealth). I detail the instruction given to both men and women before marriage, the ideas about the duties of husbands and wives, especially in relation to the care of the body, and how men and women interpreted this instruction as illustrative of their respective gendered positions. Despite men claiming the dominant role in marriage, husbands became their wives' pupils in sexual etiquette and wives resisted marriage instruction that limited their own sexual enjoyment.

In chapter 5 I foreground my exposition of contemporary married life with a brief exploration of the extensive anthropological archive concerning rural and urban marriage in Zambia. Most former students of St. Antony's struggled to perform their allotted role of "breadwinner" and to demonstrate to peers and family members that they, not their wives, made all the major decisions. Many men received an extraordinary degree of care from their wives. While I witnessed the very real affection and friendship between partners, the absence of trust in many marriages, particularly in sexual matters, was palpable. Despite their expectations that marriage would preclude other sexual relationships, most men in this study engaged in unprotected extramarital sex. The absence of communication between husbands and wives, despite many wives' fears that their husbands would give them AIDS, was a familiar pattern. Most wives felt they could not speak, and few felt they could escape from their marriages.[16]

Chapter 6 offers insights into former students' understandings of sex and sexuality and their moral assessments. Many men identified sexuality as a site of difference between "Africans" and "Europeans."[17] They variously evaluated "African sexuality" as either superior to, or inferior to, "European sexuality." The concept of "tradition" was employed to suggest what was authentically African. Along with tradition, the Bible was invoked as the moral arbiter of sexual acts. I map out men's reported experience and discuss their sexual preferences in order to draw attention to the relevance of their sexual practices for HIV transmission. Most former students offered a hydraulic model of African male sexuality that sought regular "relief" in penetrative intercourse. Performance anxiety, evident in youthful sexual activity, continued to haunt many men in their adult lives.

Chapter 7 first discusses former students' religious understandings over a life course. I analyze their ideas about God, evil, and witchcraft, as they reflected upon their embodied experience, in order to foreground the significance of these for their responses to AIDS. All claimed belief in God, the creator of the world and all that is in it. According to many students, God both helped and punished human beings in this life. While all self-identified as Christians, and many of them Catholics, few professed adherence to the major tenets of Christianity. Many students spoke of their fear of witchcraft because of the "jealousy," that is envy, that they considered to be a "natural" capacity of all "Africans." I detected some continuities over the twenty-year period in their religious understandings. For example, many men's youthful preference for the creation story of Genesis and their rejection of the theory of evolution endured. A degree of polarization had also taken place. For example, several men had become even more skeptical about many aspects of Christian teaching than they had been formerly, especially with regard to the notion of an afterlife. In contrast, a few of them had had a conversion experience, becoming Born Again and joining a Pentecostal church, or had returned to the church of their youth with renewed conviction. While few former students attended religious services, many resorted to "Christianity," as they did to "tradition," to bolster their claims of male "superiority." I describe how men and their wives, in their grief and loss, strove to understand the HIV/AIDS pandemic in the context of their religious understandings of human experience. "Has God come in another way?" some wondered. "Can faith in God cure AIDS?" I explore the relevance of former students' religious practice for their sexual conduct. Confronted with the deaths of family and friends, witchcraft remained available as an explanatory discourse for some men.

In chapter 8, I discuss responses of former students and their wives toward HIV-prevention campaigns where "sex" is constructed as a particular kind of "moral object" (Pigg and Adams 2005). I outline evaluations of prevention campaigns with their Abstain, Be Faithful, Use a Condom (ABC) messages, and of treatment campaigns that encouraged testing for HIV. Despite their own continuing extramarital (and usually unprotected) sexual activity, most men, like their wives, denounced the promotion of condoms as the encouragement to engage in "promiscuous" and "immoral" behavior. Parents wondered what they should tell their children about the best protection against HIV; most considered abstinence to be the only viable solution. I interrogate the continuing reluctance of both men and women to attend Voluntary Counseling and Testing (VCT) centers to discover their HIV status despite the increasing availability of antiretroviral therapy. Men trusted that tradition would protect them from their wives' desire that their husbands should have an HIV test. There was little space in campaigns to explore the terrain on which sexual relationships were acted out or to challenge the prevailing gender order.

The conclusion, chapter 9, positions this group of mostly elite Zambians within the context of the HIV/AIDS crisis. I draw attention to the gap between many men's attempts to perform as "real men" and their private recognition of the artifice entailed in such performances. I explore the potential of educational programs that utilize process drama techniques to create the space for the exploration of the multiple complex issues that the pandemic raises. Key to this potential is the opportunity process drama offers to explore alternative modes of being in the subjunctive mood and to promote empathy among, and between, boys and girls, men and women, differently and inequitably situated in contemporary Africa.

HIV/AIDS has brought particular challenges to the hegemonic construction of heterosexual masculinity in Zambia. This study demonstrates that, even within a small group of former mission school students, men are variously positioned in relation to this construction, some contesting it and maintaining a greater distance from it than others. I argue that many more might be ready to challenge dangerous ideologies of masculinity. This offers hope for continuing efforts to combat the pandemic in Africa.

2

Fathers and Sons:
The Measure of a Man

In a man's retelling of his childhood, it was his father—usually described as a silent, emotionally distant figure—who set the measure for his son of what it meant to be a "real man," a position most boys strove earnestly to attain. While highlighting the role of the father, I recognize the need to go beyond the Oedipal triangle of mother and father and to acknowledge the contributions of many women—not least sisters—and men to a boy's education in manhood.[1] There was a marked consistency between the narratives of childhood relationships with fathers first given to me in the men's late teens and again twenty years later. Memory is constantly being constructed, but what was striking was that although the details of a father's training in discipline remained the same, the moral evaluation of that training had shifted to become a wholly positive one.

Many former students said they remembered little about their early childhood. For some there was an enduring early image in memory, the significance of the event apparently unrecoverable. Paul recalled walking with his father around the age of three or four to visit his father's male friend, admiring the friend's way of standing and desiring to imitate it. Many men recalled distinct emotions or events, though they were unable to date them with any accuracy. For some a tragic incident remained painfully etched upon the memory: a baby brother who drowned, having fallen from his mother's back while she was crossing a bridge above a river swollen by heavy rains; an older five-year-old sister—a nursemaid—killed in a road accident; an older brother dying in a fire when the boy was five years old. Some men wept as they sorrowfully relived the pain of losing family members. Other memories were recalled with pleasure: a father's gift of clothes on his return after a prolonged absence, or for Christmas or a birthday, shone out as a beacon upon this time.

Men almost unanimously characterized the relationship between a father and a son during childhood and adolescence as a difficult one. From an adolescent son's perspective, his relationship with his father was, at best, ambivalent, because of his fear of him. Paul described having such fear of his father, a youth worker, and yet commented, "I desperately wanted to love and honor him." Distance between a man and his son was, former students said, "normal in African families." Birth order, however, was often a significant factor in the tenor of the relationship both in boyhood and in later life. The conduct and behavior of first-born sons received very particular paternal scrutiny, to be explained perhaps in part by the fact that the first-born son was expected to become the "father" of his siblings when his father died.[2] Emotional distance evaporated with younger siblings as the father grew older; the relationship between the youngest son and the aging father became more like that between grandfather and grandson, a joking relationship in which both parties enjoyed a considerable degree of familiarity. Older sons, however, strove to maintain distance, keeping as far out of their fathers' path as possible. Work took fathers away from the home either on a daily basis or caused them to be absent for months at a time. In rural households, boys accompanied their fathers in hunting and fishing, though this became less common once the child started school. Beer drinking also often took fathers away from the household, both at night and during a child's waking hours. It was when fathers were drunk that they were at their most brutal, quick to strike out against a boy, his siblings, and his mother.

The distance of "respect" demanded by adult men meant that sons at times felt they knew little about their fathers—a cause for regret for those who lost their fathers at an early age. What the men experienced as the absence of emotional warmth and physical affection from their fathers, once past infancy, was often contrasted with the supposed warmth and affection that white fathers were thought to give their children. As adolescents, former students cited instances witnessed in towns or scenes from television that depicted fathers hugging boys and young adults, commenting, "You Europeans really love your children!" Many respondents were uncertain whether to describe their adolescent feelings toward their fathers as those of respect or fear, though most came down on the side of fear. Part of the problem for the ethnographer is that the two concepts are inextricably intertwined in the vernacular expressions former students used to encapsulate the essence of the father-son relationship—in Bemba *umucinshi*, in Tonga *bulemu*—and carry both connotations on a sliding scale.

This contrasted sharply with the close relationship with his mother normally described by a son, even though in the early years she was usually the one to exercise corporal punishment. Almost all men recalled an emotional closeness to their mothers when they were children. This close tie, men said, remained in adulthood, revealing that they were more trusting of their mothers than of their wives and other sexual partners. In their ethnographies of rural marriage and family life, both Richards on the Bemba and Colson on the Tonga have remarked upon the enduring closeness and affection between a mother and her son.[3] Other commentators on Zambian family life have contended that the "unsatisfactory" resolution of the weaning crisis might well explain later marital difficulties.[4] In the mother-son relationship described by this cohort, however, there was no evidence of the conscious resentment, at least toward the mother, that one might expect to find because of the alleged trauma of abrupt weaning after being fed on demand. Exceptionally, when a son expressed resentment toward his mother, it was because the boy had felt rejected by her, when they were separated because of divorce or because of the mother's absence from home through work, training, or study. Stepmothers, however, figured prominently in memory as cruel, at times disrupting a boy's already fragile relationship with the father, though at times strengthening it. Paul's father brought another woman into the household when his mother left for studies. He told Paul that he should call her "Mother." Though Paul wanted to be friends with her, he found her to be very harsh. He recalled:

> I think also there was an element of cruelty in her disposition, so I think, well, most of the problems arose in her treatment of my younger sisters.... She used to mete out physical punishment and she used to hide the food, hide the good food. I took it for granted that there was no money or whatever, but strangely, every time dad comes back home, there used to be all sorts of funny foods to go with the occasion. She had a habit of hiding the bread, even until some of the bread got stale, and then putting it in the kitchen for us to eat. Then she would buy fresh bread and hide it again. So I grew up thinking that bread was not a very pleasant food. There was always this stale smell; it took me a long time to realize that you could also have this bread fresh. The other thing, I think as time went on, even though I had been neutral toward her, she started coming on to me in a very strange manner. She became abusive—both in the way she talked and the way she curtailed my freedom and the way she tried to beat me, until one time, just a few months before she left, I was sitting next to her outside the house around this time, around seventeen-thirty. We had the habit of sitting

around the house. There was a little platform. It was slightly high, so you could sit comfortably. And she would probably be preparing some dry foods. She was actually cooking outside. And I was sitting playing with a plank. I was hitting it on the ground. I think she got so irritated. She didn't say anything. She just took it out of my hand and hammered the plank right in the middle of my head. For the first time in my life I really did rebel because I remember I grabbed the plank from her and I wanted to hit her. And if she had not closed the door, it would have been a totally different story because at that time I was slightly bigger. I wasn't a man yet, but I was a big boy and I was getting stronger. I was in grade four. I was ten or eleven years old. So I think that was the very last picture I have of her.

Boys' Work and Play

There were differences in the chores which boys and girls were required to do in or around the household. The designation of chores revealed explicit ideas about gender-appropriate tasks. Earlier ethnographers described aspects of childhood play at around the ages of five or six that closely mimicked the adult world. Colson (1958) noted that young children acted out the particular type of work associated with each sex in the Tonga game known as *mantomba*—the boys building shelters, the girls preparing food. Colson observed, "The fact that they emphasize the difference in masculine and feminine activities shows how deeply it has already become a part of their general acceptance of what is right and proper" (1958: 261). She was unsure about the degree of early sexual experimentation. Former students, especially those who grew up in rural areas, recalled such games with their gender-appropriate roles but invariably associated such play with early sexual knowledge. Imitation of the adult world always meant the boys taking on the role of husband.

Men recalled that decisions about work tended to rest with their fathers. Any departure from what was generally judged appropriate duties for men and women was signaled by a father's willingness to perform "womanly" tasks such as cleaning the home, cooking, and washing dishes. A father's willingness to engage in "women's work" appeared to have had an impact upon those men who saw this and who, in their turn as husbands and fathers, took at least some share in indoor household jobs and childcare. Mutinta, for example, recalled his father sharing childcare and regularly washing up after meals. Mutinta and his brothers thought nothing of being expected to do their share of washing and cleaning. Such men were also the ones—the minority—who expressed a desire for at least a measure of equality between husband and wife.[5] Allocation of tasks depended in part upon the number and gender of siblings within the household. Where sisters or other girls were present they were expected to assist their mothers in the "feminine" tasks of collecting and heating water, washing, cleaning, and cooking. Where there were only male children, or where the majority were males, outcomes varied. In some of these households, boys were told to undertake these tasks; in others, said to be "very traditional," fathers forbade their sons to engage in activities apparently considered to have the potential to emasculate. Kangwa, the first-born in his family, said he and his seven brothers "felt fine" about leaving all the housework to their mother and only sister.

Boys of cattle-keeping fathers were given herding responsibilities at a young age. These tasks were explicitly described—by fathers to sons and by respondents to me—as training in manhood. They afforded the boys an escape from parental surveillance. Men happily recalled days of wandering through the bush, picking wild fruits, killing birds with their catapults, hunting duikers and porcupines, swimming and impromptu games of football called *chipombwa*—in which the ball was made from pieces of plastic bags wrapped tightly together and tied with bark or string. Some said they were reluctant to forsake this freedom for the discipline of school life. There was the new challenge of establishing one's position among the gang of boys also entrusted with herding duties. A prime peer-group value was physical strength, exhibited in the way a boy handled the animals in his charge, but what was also demanded of him was evidence of fighting prowess. Early in life, violence became an affirmation of manhood. One's place in the pecking order of the boys' gang was determined by the outcome of physical struggle. Boys were made to fight by older boys. The victor won from them the right to be exempted from work. Hambayi recalled how his father had told him that a Tonga man with no cattle was no man at all. At the age of six, he was sent with the other herdboys in his village and described how he grew in strength, becoming a skilful fighter who was able to control cattle:

> We used to look after cattle with older boys. We younger ones would refuse to go and bring back stray cattle from crop fields. An older person would go and do that and when he came back he would make us younger ones fight. He would tell us that the loser will be the one controlling animals so that they don't stray. I became strong by the age of nine through fighting. That's how I developed my physical strength.

Not all the boys readily accepted this pugilistic regime. Those who fell into this category were generally also the ones who delayed their sexual debut until their late teens or early twenties, or exceptionally, like Peter, a member of the Seventh Day Adventist Church, until marriage. He recalled, at thirty-seven: "Sometimes the bigger boys would make the bulls from different villages to fight, and then the dogs, and then the smaller boys. I had to undergo all that. I never liked fighting. I easily cried. Immediately I lost my temper I would cry. Somebody would be slapping me in the face, I would only cry."

Urban childhood also required that boys develop fighting skills to defend themselves or to mark out with other boys their gang's territory and defend it. Paul took up karate in order to withstand his father's beatings and the cruelty of his stepmother but also to fend for himself, in the absence of his older brothers, on the streets of the Copperbelt town where he grew up. He described how fighting skills and "toughness" were also inculcated by his father, though he recalled times when he realized that discretion was the better part of valor:

> My father had a philosophy: if you were beaten by somebody, then you had to go and [take] revenge. He would never allow you to cry—you know, in front of his house. If he found you crying, "What are you crying about?"—That's my father. "It's that bigger boy! He beat me!" "Go back right now and do what he did to you, back to him, and then come back again." But if he was too big (laughing), you know, you'd go behind the house and behind the trees and then come back again. (Laughing.) "What has happened?" "Yes, I've revenged! I've whipped him!" (laughing). He'd say, "Yeah—that's right! Now you can sit!"

Most of the cohort remembered older boys, mentors, whose physique and fighting skills they admired unreservedly, and who protected them from bullies. Paul's first mentor was his cousin, a skilled fighter whose ambition was to be a professional boxer. In grade five Paul had another mentor, one year older than himself, whom he recalled, he "absolutely admired" because he appeared to be so "cool." It was the boy's powerful bodily presence that attracted Paul. His friend was shorter than he was but stocky in build and an accomplished boxer. Hambayi recalled that no boy dared to lay a finger on him at primary school, protected as he was by his mentor. A mentor not only shielded his protégé but he also instructed him in the art of approaching girls, often preparing the girls in advance. The growing ability to fight and to defend oneself was associated with increasing confidence to approach girls for sex.

Father's Discipline

Training for adult life involved learning discipline. An important method of a father's discipline was physical punishment. Beyond the pain and shame experienced when a father punished his son in this way, the boy was offered certain lessons about the way an adult man conducted himself in relation to his children (and his wife) from whom respect was demanded in recognition of the father's superior status. This is not to suggest that *all* sons in their turn expressed themselves in a similar manner toward wife and children. Paul and Peter, both of whom suffered violence at their father's hands, gave no indication of following in their father's footsteps in this regard. Nevertheless, episodes of a father's physical punishment—and the almost constant threat of it—played a crucial role in many boys' growing awareness of the meaning and the expression of manhood. A father's actions toward his son expressed his power over him and indeed his "ownership" of him, his siblings, and his mother.[6] Fathers generally stopped beating their sons when they reached their mid- or late teens. Sons noted that by then their father's strength was beginning to wane. It was also, of course, the period when they themselves, while still economically dependent, were reaching the height of their strength and vitality. Very early in their lives these boys discovered that, in the prevailing hegemonic discourse, "real men" claimed "superiority" over women and expressed this, in part, by exhibiting strength—at times in verbal and physical violence and in the repression of emotional expression. Such instruction in masculine force combined with a boy's education by his peers played a key role in the production of many men's sexual identity and in their assertions of sexual virility.

Most former students explicitly described their ability to withstand their fathers' physical punishment as part of their apprenticeship in masculine strength. They described the almost habitual harshness of their fathers, especially in their early adolescence. Sons depicted fathers as "violent," "brutal," "rough," "harsh," and "fierce." A father's beatings were always remembered as more severe than a mother's, though neither was portrayed as mere tokens of disapproval.[7] Many boys witnessed their fathers beating their mothers during arguments or in drunken brawls.[8] Kangwa vividly recalled the sorrow he felt seeing his father beating his mother. He had chosen to go to a secondary boarding school, he explained, to escape from him. At his mother's suggestion, even in the school holidays he did not reside in the household his father, a council worker, shared with Kangwa's siblings and his mother who had a stall in a local market. Kangwa, at twenty, had explained that he lived with his cousin to avoid getting drawn into quarrels and fights between his parents:

> Often my father goes and drinks a lot and then there are domestic quarrels and then, when my mother is right, I just have to tell him the truth. And for that he doesn't like me.... Even recently, he tried to beat me up and even myself, I've lost control, I've lost my temper with him. So, like now, now I am a bit big, well, I don't know what I am supposed to do when he starts challenging me. Well, let me tell the truth. The truth is I have never liked to stay with my father for a long time. It doesn't mean that he doesn't like me. He likes me! But I don't like his ways.

Twenty years later, Kangwa spoke of how his relationship with his father had improved. They had become "very good friends" in the years prior to his father's death in the early 1990s. Kangwa felt he had come to understand his father and he expressed no bitterness toward him. In his opinion his father's treatment of his mother was typical of men of his father's generation:

> My father used to hit my mother and here, well, it seems to be accepted here in Zambia. He only beat her when he was drunk. But among the older generation it was common for a man to beat his wife, but now, well, it's changing. I think it is changing among our generation because of widespread access to education. I think before men saw it as their right to beat their wives. Well, I think, in general in Zambia it is believed that a woman does belong to the household and does belong to the husband, meaning that her position in the household is low, almost as low as that of children. And then, in some groups, so much money is paid to get a woman, a wife, so they almost become possessions of the husband.

Paul recalled violent arguments and fights between his parents when he was around the age of thirteen. He spoke of his sense of helplessness as, fearful for his mother's safety, he would go in search of adults who might intervene: "I used to get completely distressed. When there was this kind of pressure at home. I would take my bicycle to go and call someone whom dad respected. I would call them and they would come and then there would be some calm for a while. It was always very painful for me. I just couldn't stand it."

At school, in class discussions with me about violence toward women, some students had regularly defended what they saw as their right to beat a future wife—their *own* wife—but not other men's wives because they did not belong to them. Twenty years later, several members of the cohort reluctantly described physically attacking their wives in the heat of a disagreement, in moments of jealous rage, out of frustration, or when drunk. They were reluctant to discuss the incidents in any great detail. They told me that they had later regretted their actions, though Darius explained this was only because he feared imprisonment. Others, like Promise, said, even boasted, that they had never used or threatened violence against their wives or other sexual partners, though some had no compunction about a "prostitute" getting hurt in the process of giving them sexual services.

Reflections on childhood such as "You were brought up with a stick" were common. Harold, the sixth-born in his family, who would later die of what was assumed to be AIDS, recalled his fear of his father, a fear quite frequently expressed among the cohort and their contemporaries: "I was very afraid of my father when I was young. Usually in those days, they'd tell me, 'Your father has come' and I'd stop being playful or whatever I was doing." Harold carried on his body a memento of his father's wrath:

> When I look back, well, of all the boys in our family, I am the one he has beaten the most.... I used to go off and play and come home late at night and he didn't like it so he beat me. He even burnt me once. He took a piece of burning wood out of the fire and beat me and it burnt me here in my stomach [pointing to a scar]. Well, he was quite drunk at the time. Both my parents drink, but he was trying to ask me where I had been when I came home late one weekend. And then I fumbled [failed to answer coherently] and he got angry and he got a piece of wood. He really hurt me. At times I would feel that I had been wrong and therefore it was all right to beat me, but at times I would feel that it was quite unfair. Of course, I couldn't tell him. He stopped beating me when I was fifteen. I was changing and working hard. It was just part of life. I love my father very much.

A father's physical punishment was also recalled as emotionally distressing, as much in unanticipated slaps as in staged moments of punishment in the presence of others. Many respondents were upset by the words of rebuke their fathers chose and the tone they used to address them. Paul, at eighteen, had commented that his father, like other "African fathers," "underrated" their sons. Nearing forty, he recalled how his father used to "observe" his children, especially his sons. Paul described his childhood fear that his father would "jump on him" at any moment. Like the majority of the cohort's fathers, Paul's father was now dead. He described him as "a good hardworking man." Paul recounted numerous occasions throughout his childhood and early adolescence when he was "beaten," "flogged," and "slapped" by his father, often in the presence of siblings and peers—which made the punishment all the more difficult to bear, especially when he judged the beating to be unjust:

> He beat me a lot! It's not that I didn't do wrong things—I did, of course.... He didn't inflict permanent injury—but it would be quite painful and it would be done in such a way that emotionally you could be devastated—because sometimes he would slap you right there on the spot—like he would call you, "What is this?" By the time I was in grade four, I'd got quite immune to the beatings. When he'd say, "It's time for a beating!" I'd get my strokes. I'd look away. I wouldn't touch my buttocks and I would walk away and go and sit and not even cry because, I think, it became meaningless. Strangely enough, every time he came back home, he would try and find a reason to beat you. I mean he would search you out, until he found a reason—terrible beatings. I mean it wasn't just for me at some point. The discipline extended to all the older boys in the family.

Promise, thirty-seven in 2002, the first-born of his father's children, recounted several occasions when he felt the pain of his father's wrath:

> Up to now, my father is a very, very tough man. We children never used to associate with him, but we were very much with my mother. As a family we used to fear him. He was rough, really rough! He never used to beat anyhow, that was the good thing, but when he touched you! I remember at one time, when I was in grade four, well, I was fond of beating my sister. I cannot forget. He got a knife. He took me in the bathroom and said: "So, it seems to be a tendency with you. Now I will kill you! After killing you, I will kill myself!" Then he got hold of the sharp part of the knife. Then with the blunt end, he started beating me on the head. Beating, beating—all over the head. The whole head was swollen for a week. I was even admitted to hospital. Mother came crying, trying to intervene, because it looked like he was going to—well, according to what he was saying, "He is giving me problems!" He was a violent man, especially towards his family.

In conversation with me, Promise's father said he could not remember any of this. He said he had never had to beat Promise as he was very obedient and hardworking. He was unable to recall an incident when, according to Promise and other family members, he had escorted his son back to boarding school at gunpoint after Promise had absconded to spend time with a girlfriend.

Several members of the cohort in turn used physical punishment on their own sons, though beating daughters, once past infancy, they told me, was "taboo."[9] Neither Paul nor Peter beat their sons. However, Hambayi and Promise did. When I asked them about this, they remarked that they felt that their own beatings "had a limit"—unlike the beatings they had at times been subjected to by their own fathers—especially when the latter were drunk. Hambayi and Promise recognized that their teenage sons were afraid of them. My own observations seemed to bear out their assessment—the boys hardly speaking in their fathers' presence and doing all they could to keep out of the way and beyond reach. When they were called by their fathers in my presence, their voice tones and pitch, gestures and body language expressed deference; many knelt, with their heads bowed, and only spoke to answer questions put to them. Some of them were clearly nervous.[10]

Some punishment directly concerned work. Colson noted that when a Tonga boy was set to work herding cattle the affection between father and son soon became subject to "severe strain" (1958: 234). Hambayi, at forty, recalled his father's punishment when as a boy of seven or eight he neglected his herding duties. In retrospect, at forty, Hambayi saw this as necessary, indeed invaluable, training for a man's life:

> My father cared about the welfare of the family. But then he had some ways of punishing us, to make us feel that life is not easy. He would say, "Okay, fine, you are looking after animals [cattle]." But if they grazed somebody's field [crops], he wouldn't let us sleep in our house. We would go into the bush. He would beat us up with the animal skin we used to tie animals with. We would be eating *nshima* [maize porridge] by the fire. He would hide the whip. When the *nshima* was about to be finished he would whip us all and we would scamper in different directions. And he would tell us, "If you are really boys, don't come to my home." We would be there in the bush for two days or so, but our mother used to care for us. We would come in the night; she would hide food for us in our room. We were two, I and my elder brother. We would sleep in the bush! In the bush, honestly. We took that as a test to make us real boys. We were immature but what he did to us helped us at [to get to] the level which I am now. I still thank him up to this time because he has educated me.

School and School Work

Most former students started their primary education between the ages of seven and nine. Some of them attended as many as five different primary schools because their fathers' work necessitated the transfer of the family to a different part of the country. Several boys failed to gain sufficiently high marks in their first attempt at the grade seven exam and so repeated the last year and sometimes the last two years of primary school in order to "pass," that is, gain entry into secondary boarding school. Some attended primary boarding schools where the discipline of the teachers was surpassed in severity by the regimes imposed by older boys, bullies, or prefects, to whose excesses teachers turned a blind eye. From the vantage point of a successful career, Henry, approaching forty, looked back upon his primary education at a boys' boarding school and concluded, "It made me." He explained that he had learnt how to "fight dirty" in order to defend himself from bullies. The daily routines he recalled as particularly tough: "We, the very small boys, were told to wake up at three in the morning and go and sweep outside. And if you didn't do your work properly, well, you were really beaten up, slapped, maybe even whipped."

Parents, especially fathers, repeatedly reminded their sons that they would not always be there. At times the question was starkly put to the child: "What will you do if we die?" Boys were warned to achieve independence as soon as they could. In contrast, parents explained that a daughter could always marry and be provided for by her husband. Acting "like a man" entailed achieving independence. This was to be done by getting academic qualifications that, in theory, would deliver a well-paid job, enabling a man to marry, provide for his wife and children, assist his parents in their old age, and help other members of his family. Boys understood going away to boarding school as the necessary preparation for being able to "stand alone" and for the achievement of the adult male role. As in the tradition of the British public school, boarding education was expected to make men of them. (See Heward 1988.) Pupils accepted a teacher's right to beat them for misdemeanors, the punishment recalled most vividly when a boy was chastised in the presence of fellow pupils and other teachers because his experience of humiliation was that much greater. Poor performance in primary school tests gave a father further cause to discipline his son. Many men in the cohort spoke of the stress they felt they were under to perform well and the beatings they received when they did not. Indeed for some fathers it appeared that nothing but the first position in class was good enough. Peter recalled the beatings he received from his father for his examination results. He described his father as "a man who liked fighting." Throughout his childhood, he had seen his father attack people without warning, repeatedly beating his mother, and even on one occasion slapping and punching Peter's male primary school teacher. Like other former students, Peter had come to think of his father, now dead, in a positive light, expressing gratitude for his painful, but, he judged, necessary lessons:

> [My father] used to beat me terribly, terribly, especially if I got more than five mathematics questions wrong. He used a belt on my buttocks. Beating always hurts. It was terrible. At that time I hated him for that, but this time when I realize that he was teaching me a very good lesson. I like him for that and I wish he was still alive. I was going to tell him frankly that he was teaching me a good lesson. The last time was when I was doing my mock exam for the grade seven exam. I was seventeen. It was just a slap because I got second position. The first was a girl, by one mark. Just there, in full view of my teachers, he slapped me. In the meantime my teachers gave me a present.

Simon spoke about the strain that he felt he was under from his father, a university graduate:

> There was that pressure that I should act more like a man and not like a girl. I should grow up to be a man. And, like, I mean my father helped me a lot with my arithmetic—in grade six and towards grade seven. He would beat me on the head with the cooking stick! (Laughing.) It wasn't just symbolic. It hurt. I think he felt that I was going to lag behind and if I didn't make it as a boy, as a man, then I would be in problems, because there is always that thing that with women, they can always get married. But with a man, you support yourself.

Difficulties occurred even in father-son relationships characterized by a degree of fondness. When criticized or scolded by their fathers, most sons reported that they had kept silent. Silence was the idiom of respect. They felt that they could not speak in their own defense and were fearful of provoking an even fiercer response should they attempt to "answer back." In exceptional cases a boy took it upon himself to argue with his father. Edmund recalled his childhood and adolescence, brought up mostly by his paternal grandmother after his mother died when he was five and his father had remarried:

> My dad and I, all along, we had our own problems. Dad was fond of me. I liked him, but then we could never stay together for too

long.... He didn't like it when I defended my brothers by justifying their actions which my father thought were wrong. At one stage he scolded me, "Why do you always want to be their lawyer?"

There *were* instances of a close relationship between father and adolescent son, not clouded by fear, but these were the exceptions. When they occurred, it was often in families where the son had also observed a measure of equality between his parents and, indeed, where a father had rejected certain stereotypically hegemonic "masculine" poses. Close father-son relationships also arose at times when a young boy's mother had died or when a child had remained with his father following his parents' separation or divorce. It is striking that former students refrained from explicit censure of their fathers' extramarital relationships that often caused the divorce. Other periods of a son's separation from his mother were caused by a mother's absence because of study and work, or because of childbirth or illness. While men in these cases recalled the early pain of separation from the mother, several describing it as "torture," some described how fathers became "mothers," that is, gentle and affectionate, in their caring attention.

At nineteen, Leonard, the third-born in his family, who would later die from what was assumed to be AIDS, explained the unusually close relationship he enjoyed with his father:

> I feel closer to my father than to my mother. Maybe it's because of the way I was brought up, because when I was born, two weeks passed and then my mother was admitted to hospital and she had to be isolated. Up to now I don't really know what the problem was. She was in Lusaka and dad had to take me to Eastern Province. She only came home to find me when I had already started walking. That's what they tell me—I don't remember any of this because I was too young. I think I am closer to my dad because of what happened when I was born and also dad continued to pay a lot of attention to me even when I was older. He would always call me, talk to me. We'd always have chats together. He rarely did that with the others.

Absent Fathers

Men who had had to grow up *without* a father nearby expressed bitterness. This was most usually because the son felt he had been abandoned and left without a father's physical protection and material support, even though in several households it was the mother's contribution, often raising money through brewing and selling beer, that had enabled a boy to go to school. At nineteen, Sampa, who had last seen his father seven years prior to our discussion, explained his feelings:

> My father took my mother when he was already married to the niece of my grandfather. When my mother came to see my grandfather, things went berserk. Then my mother became pregnant. It was really bad—married to one woman and having sex with her sister. It is a bad thing! I think I would have been happy if my parents had married.

In later life, Sampa explained that he had decided it was better to keep his distance from his father because he had discovered that he was suspected of being a witch. In his thirties, Hambayi had harbored similar suspicions of his own father, explaining to me, when I had expressed my doubts, "We cannot know what is in his heart."[11] Hambayi's first wife and two of his children died. His visits to various diviners had confirmed his suspicions about his father's involvement in their deaths. The past and past relationships, however, were open to revision. At forty, and with his father now dead, Hambayi concluded that he would not have acted in this way toward him and his family.

In spite of a boy's fear of his father, his temporary absences from the household might create apprehension in a son and other family members because of the quotidian threat of thieves, especially in urban areas. Although Paul had lived in fear of his father, he vividly recalled feeling unprotected when his father was away:

> There was always that sense of insecurity because my father used to go away for long periods of time. What if a thief came at home? You used to hear footsteps outside the house, "What's that?" My heart would be pumping. You'd be—I'd be just watching. There were these orange streetlights which would easily cast a shadow if someone passed near the house. I'd be watching for a shadow, wondering what would happen next. So we learnt to sleep with weapons under our bed, me and my elder brother, you know, to defend ourselves.

Joshua's father had died when he was an infant. His ailing mother had not remarried. He, too, had been anxious about thieves and about the fact that his mother had no adult support in the home. Indeed, Joshua attributed what he considered his lack of "manly" characteristics to the absence of a father figure. He agreed with other men and women who said that he "acted like a woman," even though as a married man with several children he had achieved adult status and a prominent position in his town and within his church. He explained:

> I think not having a father contributed to the element of fear that I always had. When we were children, my mother was living alone with us. A few times thieves broke into our home; neighbors fought over land and so on and over children's behavior. My mother stood up to the families that came with their husbands to complain about what my sister may have done or the son may have done. As a child I could not run to somebody when I saw my mother being confronted. That has made me believe that if there had been a man in the home I would have been a more formidable character. I say to my children that had my father and mother lived on, I would have been much better—a better person, a stronger person, much more decisive. My character is not confrontational. Had my father been around I probably would have learnt to fight and even handle a gun much earlier.

Conclusion

The tenor of most Zambian father-son relationships during a son's childhood and adolescence is best described as a relationship of fear and emotional distance. In his analysis of customary ideas of manliness in Zambia's lower Zambezi valley, Dover, commenting that the "traditional" Chiawa father figure should be "'feared' and obeyed" (2001: 95), observes, "Emotional succour is given by fathers to small children, but with older offspring there should be a relationship of respect" (ibid.: 139).

For former students, this relationship altered during the life-course when fathers became "good friends" with sons who had surpassed them in vigor and often in material wealth. After a father's death, sons spoke of their warm appreciation for the discipline their fathers had meted out to them. Perhaps this was out of compassion and empathy, or because the son, in achieving the status of husband and father in his turn, now wished to claim for himself the privileges that he had seen his father enjoy.

It is striking that, reflecting as adults upon their upbringing, these men unanimously expressed gratitude toward their fathers for the punishment they had received at their hands. They described this training as formative and were ready to overlook instances of a father's unjust punishment, especially when he was drunk. How should we interpret the absence of any expressions of resentment? Was this merely the extension of the respect due to elders? Was it the result of the forgiving and tolerant attitude that many men held as an important human value? Or would the depiction of a disreputable father by an unforgiving son reflect too painfully and shamefully upon the teller both in his own eyes and in the eyes of others? Perhaps for men whose fathers were now dead there was no desire, indeed perhaps an unspoken fear, to speak ill of the dead. Dead fathers, for some men, continued to exist and were thought to dwell not far from the living.

Some former students, as adults, would draw upon the model of a silent, harsh father and husband, a man among men. In memory, a man's father could become an exemplar of how to behave toward his own wife and children and of what to demand from them, as well as how to conduct sexual relationships with other women. Yet many boys, like Kangwa and Paul, had witnessed the violence their mothers suffered at their fathers' hands. They had felt helpless in their failure to protect the person whom they felt closest to in the whole world. The Zambia Demographic and Health Survey 2001–2002 (Central Statistical Office of Zambia 2003) suggests that such violence is in no way unusual. In this nationally representative survey of 7,658 women (15–49 yrs), more than half reported having experienced beatings or physical mistreatment since the age of 15, and 24 percent had experienced physical violence in the 12 months preceding the survey. The survey claims, "Among physically abused women currently in union, almost eight in ten report their current husband/partner as a perpetrator of the violence" (Central Statistical Office of Zambia 2003: xxiv). Of all the women surveyed, 85 percent stated that they believed that a husband might have justifiable cause to beat his wife, 52 percent of these citing arguing with a husband, and 86 percent citing a wife having an extramarital partner, as sufficient causes.

All the men in this study felt they had to struggle as boys under the paternal gaze and among their peers to achieve manhood. As men, the expression of male sexual identity was often figured as an inherently violent activity in which, in competition with other men, the conquest of women was the central element. This entailed, for the majority, unprotected sexual intercourse with multiple partners. For many men, childhood and adolescent lessons in manliness would militate against their playing a positive role in the prevention of HIV/AIDS. The abiding legacy of their instruction in masculinity placed former students and those they had sex with at increased risk, as I demonstrate in the following chapters.

3

LEARNING SEX IN AND OUT OF SCHOOL

Many men recalled games from the age of five or six, before they started school, which involved the exploration of girls' bodies, and, for some, boys' bodies as well, and attempts to imitate the heterosexual behavior of adults.[1] Men would later differentiate this play activity from their first "real" experience of sex, as Darius explained:

> I sort of had sex with small girls before I went to primary school, but I can't remember much about it. We would pair off and try to have sex, but that sex is different from the sex I know now. At that time I wouldn't release sperms. I would just push my penis into the girl. But nothing would happen. I wouldn't feel any relief. I think it was because I was too young.

Several men described seeing older boys and adults, often older, male siblings and uncles, engaged in sexual intercourse. None of the men interviewed spoke of seeing their parents having intercourse. They may well not have done so, or the taboos around witnessing such an event may have prevented its being reported or the memory might well have been repressed. Christopher recalled his rural childhood and his earliest sexual experiences in the context of play:

> I would say that I learnt about sex like other kids. I just found that I knew it.... You know, in the villages in the evenings when it was starting to get dark, as kids we would play games. There would be some big boys and girls and some younger boys and girls in the group. The bigger boys would say, "Let's make some shelters!" And then they'd say, "Ok, this is your wife and this is my wife, and so on. Then they'd say, 'We'll go and sleep now.'" And maybe they'd say, "The little ones will be dogs and cocks." Now you who were dogs and cocks you would see what was happening. They would know you were watching them. They would do the act and you would see, so, now, as you became

big—big in your mind I mean—you would also try to do it with your age-mates. Maybe you'd steal some mealie-meal from home. You see, then, you'd be just like people at home in a village.

What was important to the boys was that they should lie on top of the girls. From an early age boys understood that they were required to assert the active role, spatially expressed as "above," and the girl should take the passive role—"below" in the encounter.[2] Enoch dated his initial awareness about sex to the time he started primary school at seven. Grade one classmates boys and girls would pair off, girls saying, "This is my husband" and boys saying, "This is my wife." Comments such as "You and your wife," by which his mother and his aunts referred to him and the small girls he played with, caused Kangwa to think about the relationship between men and women. He recalled games around the age of five with female cousins and other small girls:

> We used to organize some small households. You'd pretend that there is a small household here, a small household there. The boys would build the shelters. The girls would cook. There's a husband and wife and there's a husband and wife. That's how I learnt about sex.... Small children would be cockerels and they would watch the husbands and wives. We called it "cooking in small quantities." The cooking accompanies the whole thing. I mean you don't just end up cooking small quantities of *nshima* and relish. You try to pretend that you are a normal big person.

Often they did not take off their clothes. There was no penetration. It was not, as Kangwa ruefully commented later in his life and in failing health, "the kind of sex that would give you AIDS."

Parents' Silence

Richards noted that, while the Bemba discussed certain physical facts frankly, they used "a variety of euphemisms when discussing sex relations and are particularly careful when members of different age groups are present" (1969: 17).[3] Almost all students reported that it was taboo for parents to speak to their sons about sex, though Dominic's mother recommended local medicine to increase his sexual potency. (Many married men later reported the pressure they felt, especially from their mothers, to produce children.) For the most part a discreet silence was maintained on both sides. While this silence fitted prevailing notions of "respect" and propriety, many men regretted that while instruction in sexual matters was given to their sisters at puberty and again prior to marriage, they were left to find out for themselves. (Dover similarly describes contemporary teaching for boys about sexuality among the Goba in southern Zambia as "haphazard" [2001: 106].)

When a younger sibling was born, parents had told small boys that they had bought the baby at ZCBC (a supermarket). Most parents made oblique allusions to discourage their young son from sexual activity, which would distract him from his studies, and, should it result in a pregnancy, might cause a boy to be expelled from school. What little explicit advice was available to boys came from grandparents and uncles, though as families spread to various parts of the country few had grandmothers nearby who could whisper to them. Their main source of information was slightly older male peers who taught that "strength"—both physical and sexual—was the most important quality to attain. Sexual knowledge was generally assumed to come "naturally" to boys. Some boys were puzzled by what they learnt to call "wet dreams" and sought advice from male cousins and peers. Many recalled that, as young boys, they had been taught that sex was bad. Parents and elders told them that girls bit boys.[4] Sampa recalled specific warnings from elders: "They would tell us '*Ngamuleyangala nabanakashi mukapya*'—'If you have sex with girls, your penis will get burnt.'" Sampa's mother recalled elders warning her, when she was young, that if she had sex with boys her fingers would grow abnormally long.[5] Boys were warned that some girls had diseases and that if they got a sexually transmitted disease their penis would have to be cut off.

Incidents, which men later recalled as "sexual abuse," were rarely communicated to parents and adults. About such unreported experience, as in discussions of "homosexual" activity in Zambia, men often spoke of the "African gift of silence." Some men claimed to have been abused by older girls or women. Sampa asked me whether it was possible for a man to be raped by a woman. He described an incident around the age of eleven, before, he said, he was able to produce semen though he had already attempted penetrative intercourse with a number of girls of his own age. He was called into an outdoor shower by a "big [mature] woman," a neighbor, as he was passing:

> She was bathing. She called me, "You can you bring me some soap?" I went inside there and she did what she wanted to do with me. She made love. I was so young. I found her naked, but she said, "No, just come!" By that time I had already known these things. So I knew what

she wanted. I was ready. I had an erection. She just pulled down my shorts.

In adulthood, Darius concluded that, as children, he and his younger brother had been "sexually abused" by their sixteen-year-old cousin and stepsister who would bathe them:

> My cousin would start playing with my penis. She would just play with it. Then my stepsister did the same. She also actually played [had intercourse] with my stepbrother. They were both from the same mother and the same father. So she wanted to entice me. She would even ask to bath me. Whenever she went with my younger brother who accepted being bathed she would sort of abuse him, but the boy would come and show me what the girl was doing to him. She was masturbating him and putting his penis inside her vagina.

In his father's village, from the age of seven Hambayi had shared a hut and a makeshift bed with two male cousins who were his agemates and who herded his father's cattle with him. At least one of the threesome would slip away to spend the night with a girlfriend but in the morning when it was time for work all would be present. They looked out for one another. Attending upper primary school eight miles from home as a weekly boarder afforded Hambayi more opportunities for sexual encounters. His soccer skills attracted many girls who were willing to have sex with him.

Groups played an important role in many boys' early sexual experiences. What Enoch considered his first sexual encounter after early childhood play was around the age of ten when he was in grade four; it was in a group with three other boys from his class and it provided an early lesson in exchange:

> There was this lady, well, she must have been around eighteen. She told me and my friends, "If you buy sweets for me, I will let you have sex with me." I didn't have any money but the other boys bought some sweets and we went to her house at night. It was just getting dark—towards nineteen hours. She had given us directions. When we reached the house we went straight to the room that she told us and we found her in bed pretending to be asleep. She told us to be quiet or her father would hear us. So the first boy started playing with [having sexual intercourse with] that lady, then the second, then the third and then me. But, even if I did that, I didn't have the experience because of my penis at that time. I failed to penetrate. I didn't go inside. I didn't ejaculate. I don't know whether it was because I was too young or because of a lack of experience or out of fear. I just lay on top of her.

He did not ask his classmates about their experience with the young woman. The darkness of the room prevented him from being able to observe them, and, he hoped, from being observed. During his childhood Enoch repeatedly wondered, "Is it true that the penis can go into a woman?"

Age when penetration and ejaculation were first "achieved" varied considerably, though for the majority it occurred in the early teens while the boys were in the last years of their primary education.[6] This reported age of what is sometimes referred to by some commentators as "sexual debut" is in line with other findings in Zambia. In his research on young men's sexuality in Chiawa in Southern Zambia and in Misisi, a township in Lusaka, Ndubani (2002) suggests that most men became sexually active by their mid-teens. The extensive survey data gathered by Fetters et al. (1997) in four low-income Lusaka compounds indicate the average age of what they term "sexual initiation" was between eleven and fourteen for boys and girls. For many students of St. Antony's it was the discovery of a source of great excitement and pleasure, when, as more than one explained to me, "something mysterious happens all over your body." Men's retrospective accounts were couched in the language of conquest. They recalled feelings of "being a man," though "failure" and embarrassment were not uncommon. For some boys the first experience was neither particularly memorable nor pleasurable. Indeed it could be deeply disappointing. Mentors tried to teach their protégés and organized older, sexually experienced girls for them. Hambayi told me how older boys at primary school had instructed him in the finer points of how to "run after" girls: "They would tell me to show [that I should show them] that I am a man. When I go to meet the girl I must do something." One particular mentor in sexual matters, four years older than Hambayi, was singled out for blame by Hambayi's father for teaching him "bad manners" (having sex with girls). When Hambayi's school performance deteriorated dramatically, his father beat him and forbade him to associate with the older boy.

For all the stress in many men's narratives on a man's power and his active role and sexual strength, first sexual intercourse often cast the boy in a dependent position. The ideal of male sexual conquest had been reversed: an experienced, often older, girl had taken the initiative. While some men were reassured by the girls' expertise, their obvious greater knowledge and experience made others feel, they said, "inadequate," "incompetent," and "foolish." They were embarrassed to appear "childish" when they knew that, as "men," *they* were supposed to take the lead. Some simply did not know how to proceed.

From his early teens, Darius had gone to Sundowns (village parties) to drink beer. Even though his friends would organize a girl for him, he explained to me that he was shy and scared that he would "fail to perform": "I didn't know what to do in bed. I would touch the girl's body, touch her breasts. Then that would be the end of the story. My friends would go for sex but I couldn't." David recalled friends in grade four telling him about the sex they enjoyed with their girlfriends, but it was not until grade seven that he had sexual intercourse in a group of boys and girls at his primary boarding school: "My friends encouraged me. I went with them into the girls' dormitory. Since I didn't have a girlfriend, I was told to get one of the girls. That girl I picked knew the stuff already. She started teaching me. It was very exciting. I was sixteen but she was older than me."

Leonard described the chance nature of his first experience at the age of fifteen:

> We were walking along the road near my home—me and my two friends. It was early in the morning. Now, we met three girls. They were trying to hitchhike. The other two boys were quite experienced, so they managed to convince the girls that they should walk over to my house and have some breakfast. Mum and dad were not around. Now, these other boys were leading the way and so because they were three and we were three, I found myself picking one of the girls as well. I knew what it was all leading up to. So I had sex with one of the girls. I can't remember what my reaction was. The boys were older than me and the girls were quite a bit older—seventeen or eighteen.

At primary school, much emphasis was placed upon sport. This proved an important avenue for a boy to become recognized. A pupil's sporting abilities were always highlighted in the reference provided by a primary school head when the boy won a place in grade eight. Sport was thought to be beneficial for body and spirit, encouraging sportsmanship, healthy competition, and cooperation, while also developing a boy's skills. Sports regimes in schools played a central role in masculinizing boys' bodies as they learned "a specific combination of force and skill" (Connell 1983: 18).[7] Many boys were anxious to build their physique both to defend themselves against other boys but also to develop a body that others, especially girls, would admire. Men who had been particularly gifted in sport at school recalled that there were always a number of girls ready and willing to have sex with them. Boys who could not compete in this field, but who were good at "difficult" subjects such as mathematics and science, attracted girls who sought their assistance and who often repaid the boys with sexual favors. In a parody of the behavior of some male teachers toward female pupils in Zambia, Sampa explained his *modus operandi*, revealing like many other boys an early awareness of the play of power in sex: "Even big [older] girls liked me. Maybe it was because I was intelligent at school. I used to teach the girls different things, especially mathematics. Well, then, it was just a matter of commands: 'You, okay, let's go and do something.' The girls also wanted it."

Sampa spent his early childhood with his maternal grandparents in their village. He recalled "playing sex" from around the age of twelve or thirteen with young girls. On several occasions he was discovered by adults and reported to his grandfather who would beat him. He used to have erections but was unable to produce semen. His first "proper sex," that is when he produced semen, was with a fellow pupil at primary school—a girl who was a neighbor and "a kind of cousin." They were both fourteen. They met at night in the bush close to the village. He continued his relationship with this girl for four years (though he also had sexual intercourse with many other girls during this period). At times she would refuse him. She wanted a promise of marriage from him, while other girls did not. (When Sampa was twenty they were still friends and, according to him, she still wanted to marry him.) He went to the Copperbelt to complete his primary education there. However, he would return for holidays to his grandparents' village. He remembered one four-week holiday while he was in grade seven, when he had sexual intercourse with no less than eight girls. He attributed his attraction to his being a "townsman": "The girls in the village were just on me. They thought, 'This guy, he's from town! He's better than these guys at the village.'" At fifteen, Sampa contracted venereal disease. He was afraid he would become impotent, even die. In his distress he went to his great-grandmother who first whipped him for "playing with girls" and putting his education at risk. She then gave him "traditional medicine" and he seemed to recover.

Cross-cousins figured in many accounts as the boys' first teachers in matters of sex, though some men spoke of their first sexual encounters with parallel cousins as "a kind of incest."[8] Henry's first "adult" experience was with a female cousin. He was thirteen and it happened while he was on holiday from his primary boarding school. It did not seem particularly significant to him: "The girl gave me the lead, but also by this age I was interested." Promise recalled his first penetrative sex at the age of twelve or thirteen. It marked the end of the period of masturbation with age-mates and older boys. (See later.) He remembered how shy he and the girl who was of a similar age felt: "When I proposed that first lady, I had that fear. And it wasn't proposing as such. It was a way of—ah—I just called her. She came. She covered herself, her head. Also I was feeling shy (laughing). So I had sex with her, like that."

MUTI

Boyhood anxieties to ejaculate as quickly and as "powerfully" as possible led many to seek *muti* (medicine) for "sexual strength," a practice many continued in later adult life. Several boys and young men, especially those in the rural areas, obtained love potions and aphrodisiacs from "bush doctors" in order to attract girls.[9] Some of these medicines were cigarettes made from various roots and herbs to be smoked while chanting the name of the girl they wanted to "hook." Some worried about arousing desire that would demand to be satisfied immediately. Dominic, at forty, describing himself as "a very natural person," said he had refused to use them. In adulthood he denounced the use of *muti* as a major cause of AIDS. When he was young, Dominic's anxiety about his ability to father children was focused on the size of his penis. He recalled competitions among his male friends to see who could urinate the furthest: "Well, you see, that was in a way helping the muscles in the penis to grow strong, to develop. In my experience, the amount of semen you produce doesn't seem to matter very much. It's the size of the penis. Women like a man with a big penis. According to them, it gives them more satisfaction."

While some boys disdained the use of any aphrodisiacs, claiming they were "strong" or "energetic" enough already, many were eager to obtain them. Some preparations were composed of roots soaked in water. A boy would either drink the medicine or apply it to his penis. At primary school, Enoch was eager to enlarge his penis. A classmate gave him some roots and told him to wrap them around his penis at night:

> I did what he told me. Now the penis became swollen. There was some sort of water in the penis that made it big. My penis became sore. I couldn't even urinate straight. It was very difficult to pull the foreskin back. It was very painful. It looked as if the penis would never come to the right position again. I was very worried. Eventually, it came back to normal. I never used anything after that.

Promise recalled using ants with his friends when he was very young in an attempt to increase his sexual power:

We used to take those very small ants, the brown ones that make holes. We were told by older boys to put them onto our breasts—those small breasts, the nipples. When you put them there, they would bite you and the breasts would get swollen. Now when the breasts got swollen, they said you would have more power, more sperm.

Sexual activity was often depicted in violent imagery. The ability to "fire" or "hammer" several quick "rounds" of sex at each session became for the majority an important index of manhood. Dover records similar terminology among the Goba:

> ...the emphasis on potency and fertility is still marked in Goba society. Men say that a grandfather may ask his grandsons if they have nocturnal emissions and tell them to check the consistency of their semen, which should be thick, sticky and white. Boys may be told the importance of their first "bullets" (i.e. the first "round" of intercourse when the semen is strongest) shooting deep into the woman. Semen is thus a life-giving substance whose quality should be looked after and whose name in Goba, *urume*, can be translated as "essence of manhood." (2001: 107–108)

Students' desire for several rounds of sex partially explains the men's later preference for their women partners to be "tight and dry." (See chapter 6.)

At St. Antony's some information about sex came in biology lessons, which focused on the "mechanics" of sex. There was little about relationships and emotions, though this was discussed in religious education lessons that were compulsory in the junior school but optional in the senior grades. While many students stated that they regarded premarital sex a sin, this did not prevent them from engaging in it. A few recalled feeling guilty. Dominic dated his first sexual intercourse at sixteen. He was in grade nine and the young woman, who took the initiative, was in grade twelve—four years older and already sexually experienced. He and his friends had discussed sex at school, especially at night in their dormitory:

> Well, in the end, you say to yourself, "Let me try it!" Now there was this girl. She would come to school to visit me, bringing messages from my brother. She would bring things for me. Now, I started feeling very strange—the way she was behaving. So when I asked her, well she was very frank. She said, "You come to my home." Well, I wanted

to experiment. (Laughing.) I went to her home. So it was on a weekend. I had it but I thought I had lost something. I just had a terrible feeling.

Darius also dated his first "proper sex" at the age of sixteen when he was in grade ten. It was with a younger cousin who was visiting his village. They continued to have sex regularly for the next six months. In his account, she was the one who took the initiative. The sexual relationship continued even after they had both married. Darius explained (laughing), "Even now when we meet we become mischievous." They did not use condoms, Darius explained, because he was too excited to start trying to find some, especially in a rural area where they were difficult to obtain. He recalled the first time he ejaculated into his cousin. He did not understand what was happening. Like others, he feared that he was urinating into the girl and tried to withdraw.

A few boys' first sexual intercourse was with an inexperienced younger girl. Some former students recalled forcing girls to have sex with them when they were not to be persuaded by "sweet words." In general, the men said that no love was involved in their first efforts; many spoke of the pressure of the peer group. From his analysis of focus group discussions with young men in Chiawa, Ndubani reports similar pressure: "Sexual experience was perceived as an integral part of growing up into manhood. Men were perceived to have uncontrollable sexual desire (*nhomba*). They indicated that at one stage during adolescence, a young man must have sex, failure to which their sexuality will be doubted both by peers and some of the adult male relatives" (2002: 35). Fetters et al. point to differences between Zambian male and female adolescents in the reasons they gave for engaging in sexual activity:

> For most boys sex (and desire) is seen as a natural part of growing up. Boys also gave a number of reasons related to peer pressure, proving manhood, out of love (when you have sex the love gets stronger), or if you don't have a girlfriend your friends laugh at you. For girls in school it was curiosity, help with schoolwork, love, and/or the opportunity to earn pocket money or snacks that determined whether she wanted to have sex with the boy. They also agreed to have sex with teachers for "leakage" of exam papers and other favors from the teachers. Some girls said they had sex for pleasure, or to prove they were fertile, or to appease the[ir] boyfriends who claimed they would leave them. (1997: 5)

In former students' recollections, there was a general absence of talk of emotion at first sexual intercourse and very few descriptions of kissing and cuddling.[10] Paul was an exception. He recalled that what he wanted more than anything else was to kiss and fondle a girl and he did not find it difficult to draw the line at intercourse. He came to suspect that he disappointed a number of girls, especially the more sexually experienced ones. Unaware of condoms during his primary education, his behavior, he explained, was influenced by his fear of making a girl pregnant and of having to deal with the consequences. He dreaded having to face the responsibility and embarrassment. He did not consider making a girl pregnant "cool." At the age of twelve, Paul was warned by his father who suggested another possible way of exhibiting "strength": Paul should be "strong" enough to delay sexual intercourse until he had finished his education. Though girls at primary school would write him love letters and propose relationships— evidently girls were capable of making the first move—Paul had little interest in responding to them. His school mentor could not persuade him to experiment with a girl. Paul recalled that in grade seven, "[s]ecretly within me I didn't care one way or the other. I didn't care whether I succeeded or not in those ventures. Maybe I didn't really want to succeed, you know." In retrospect, at forty, he considered that his sexual development had lagged behind his physical development. He reflected that it was perhaps this "late" development that had protected him from what he now considered premature sexual activity and from the risk of early exposure to HIV. By the time he got to secondary school, Paul was aware that the changes in his body made him more inquisitive about what many other boys had been talking about. He became curious about girls and conscious that as a boy he was expected to take the leading role: "I understood that they were the objects that were to be conquered or to be put under your wing, or at your feet." By the end of grade eight he had made new friends, among them one he described as "a very naughty boy"—a mentor in sexual matters. This new friend kept challenging Paul's ignorance about sexual issues. He did this, Paul recalled, "in a very aggressive way. But in his way trying to get me to become the better man, the full, complete man, the man that one should be, by knowing about such things and by having the kind of experience that he claimed to have himself." Paul soon realized that a "real man" had several girlfriends and he tried to have girlfriends in different towns.

The boys and young men routinely gave their girlfriends presents. Some described this gift-giving as a way of thanking them for sex, even though they noted, "traditionally," after intercourse, a woman, especially a wife, was supposed to kneel and clap her hands to thank the man. Others did not want to link the presents with a sexual transaction, preferring to consider them as expressions of love and affection.

At primary school gifts were pens, paper, exercise books, biscuits, other food, or a small amount of money. Beyond the expression of gratitude, boys were conscious that they had to make efforts to keep a girlfriend for themselves. These were expressions of power and attempts to control their sexual partners. Kangwa, at twenty, explained: "One reason I gave my girlfriends presents is that I noticed when my partner was in need. The other reason was that I wanted to be seen to be in control of a girl in case other boys were also interested in her. There was always competition. You needed to prove that you were the right one."

However, some girls proved too demanding, wanting to be provided with Coca-Cola and to be taken to the cinema, things that Kangwa could rarely afford. Giving what men continued to call presents remained a feature of their later premarital and extramarital relationships. This pattern of exchange appears common in the region both in adolescence and adulthood. Kambou et al. (1998) describe transactional adolescent sex in peri-urban Lusaka. Kaufman and Stavrou report gift-giving among young people in Durban, associated with "sexual leverage"—the entitlement of one partner "to physical and sexual rights to the other's body" (2004: 377–378). Hunter (2002) illustrates the materiality of everyday sex in a township and an informal settlement in Kwazulu-Natal. Rejecting the simplistic label of "prostitute," he argues for a distinction to be made between sex linked to subsistence and sex linked to consumption and identifies the close association between sex and gifts as a central factor driving multiple-partnered sexual relationships. Hunter illustrates the instability of masculinities in times of economic decline in contexts where "real men" are portrayed or portray themselves as providers for women. (See also Simpson [2002] for rural Zambian primary school boys' gifts and Leclerc-Madlala [2002] for such exchange between South African youth.)

Multiple Partners and Reluctance to Use Condoms

There were no reports of condom use in first sexual intercourse and very few in adolescent sexual encounters generally. Many men said that, as students, they simply had not known about condoms or where to obtain them. Besides, there was a general consensus, maintained by the majority in adult life, that condoms reduced sexual pleasure. As young men, and in later life, many men said that they had not asked whether a female partner lost sensation and pleasure when a condom was used. The minority who did said that women also reported a reduction of pleasurable sensations. Many young men said that condoms were not "natural" and therefore should not be used. Their notion of natural was inextricably bound up with their belief that God had created the world and the human beings in it. The God of Genesis had said "Go forth and multiply" and this should have nothing artificial about it, many explained, even though most were afraid of causing pregnancy.[11]

Throughout adolescence Henry had unprotected sex, partly because of his preference to "go live" (have sex without a condom) and "chance" (risk causing pregnancy); it was also partly because, being young and *looking* young, he was unable to overcome the chagrin he imagined he would feel should he attempt to buy condoms at a chemist's shop. "Chancing" was a preferable risk to the hazard of embarrassment. There was the added problem about *how* to use condoms. Inexperienced and yet anxious to appear competent at intercourse, no one wanted this pretence to be undermined by an evident lack of familiarity with them. Kangwa never used condoms because, he explained, they "taxed" (reduced) some of the feeling and in addition they encouraged "carelessness" (that is, having unprotected intercourse frequently and with a number of partners). Besides, he had "faith" in the girls he had intercourse with. In grade eleven, he developed gonorrhea and was treated at a government clinic. It took him some time to recover. Sampa said that from the age of fifteen he had started to fear that he might make a girl pregnant. He recalled having had sex with "maybe eighteen or nineteen" primary school girls. Sampa never used condoms because, he explained, he wanted to "feel something" and because the girls he had sex with did not demand them. In retrospect he was puzzled why he had had no pregnancy cases to answer: "Maybe I was too young. Maybe it's because I didn't stick to one girl. Maybe if I had had just one girlfriend, I would have made her pregnant. I don't understand because I was producing plenty of sperm." Sampa had his second episode of venereal disease in junior secondary school. By the end of grade ten, two of his closest classmates had each fathered two children with different young women. During his senior secondary school, he had three girlfriends with whom he regularly had sex. Sampa started drinking beer in grade eleven. Consuming beer before having sex made using a condom even less likely. (Many students noted that beer, unlike marijuana (*dagga*), made them "more excited" to have sex.) In addition to the possible loss of sensation, in Sampa's experience the combination of beer and a condom meant that it would take him "too long" to ejaculate and so he preferred to "go live." Most young men were suspicious of the contraceptive pill, largely because they had heard that it could cause cancer. Sampa differed from his friends in that he supplied his girlfriends with stolen contraceptive pills. He too had heard that the pill might cause cancer, but had decided that this was "a story put out to threaten [discourage] us." The general anxiety about a link between the contraceptive pill and cancer receded in later life.

On the first few occasions when Darius had sex with a new girlfriend, he used condoms. Subsequently he did not, partly because of the loss of sensation he experienced, but also because he soon "developed faith" in the girl. Ceasing to use condoms was an affirmation of trust that the partner was "clean," free of sexually transmitted infections. The partner could be trusted. (See Manuel [2005] for similar perceptions of Mozambican secondary school students who chose not to use condoms to demonstrate trust and love.) This became a familiar pattern in men's adult extramarital relationships. Many schoolboys, like Hambayi, associated condoms with "prostitution" and its promotion. He never used condoms. In his early teens, while still at primary school, he became ill, vomiting black bile. Hambayi pondered over the two explanations that older people in the village offered him. The first was that his illness was caused by witchcraft; the second was that it was the result of having sex with a woman during her menstruation. Elders explained that a woman's discharge of blood was dirty and hence could make a man ill. Although Hambayi could see no link between his sickness and his partner's period, he drank the two types of medicine his father prepared from roots and soon recovered. In secondary school, Hambayi's skepticism about the village elders' diagnosis was confirmed. His Zambian biology teacher explained to him that a woman's monthly discharge was not capable of causing sickness. However, he encouraged Hambayi and the rest of the class to leave women free from sex at this time.

Their antipathy toward condoms caused many young men to alternate frequently between partners. They judged that the longer a relationship lasted, and the more accustomed to, and eager, the boy became for regular sex, the greater the risk of causing a pregnancy. By having two or three concurrent girlfriends, a young man felt he could protect himself from this risk. As the girls would have different "safe periods," the young man felt he was free to have sex with at least one of the girls at any particular time. For many young men, if someone was using condoms it meant then that his sexual activity was excessive. By relying upon the "safe period," the boys placed the responsibility upon the girl—the extra burden of particular knowledge of the workings of her body, which had to be tamed and domesticated for male pleasure and satisfaction. Chimbala's first penetrative sex, when he was sixteen, while in grade nine, took place in a dark alley outside a disco in town on the day schools closed for the holidays. At twenty, he said he had never used a condom, but relied on the "safe period": "At one time I had three girlfriends at the same time. They didn't know about one another. I was frightened of possible pregnancies. I always check the girl's period and make sure that the girl is mature and that she knows her own body. If she says, 'No, I'm not alright,' then I leave her alone."

The number of sexual partners, especially in concurrent relationships, rapidly became for some students the measure of their achievement of manhood. In his last year at St. Antony's, Henry had two girlfriends with whom he had sex. The girls knew about one another but were each prepared to continue the relationship. In adulthood, Henry commented to me, "I explained to them that being in a boarding school meant there was a shortage of girls and so naturally I wouldn't want to turn anyone away." He recognized a double standard in his inability to accept a girlfriend who had sex with other men, attributing his feelings to "male selfishness." However, other boys explained that a girl might also leave them for another boy if she discovered that she was not his only sexual partner. In their teenage years few spoke about having the experience of falling in love and hardly any thought that such an experience was a sound basis for marriage.[12] In later life most men would dismiss their early sexual encounters as insignificant, though they vividly and excitedly recalled them.

At St. Antony's, boys preferred to have partners from what they considered the same "class," that is girls at secondary schools, and, even better, at mission schools. The most sought-after girls were convent-educated. As a secondary school student, Edmund had never used condoms.[13] AIDS was not yet on his horizon, and as to the risks of pregnancy or venereal disease, he observed the following at thirty-eight:

> The fear of pregnancy was never there until it happened. On two occasions I was said to have made a girl pregnant, but I don't believe it was

me. The risk of contracting a venereal disease from a girlfriend was very slim, unless one went to a prostitute. But those days I used to be conscious of class. It wasn't a question of a girl's beauty. We had a clique of girls—a few notables you could go out with. So the question of venereal diseases did not arise.

Almost half the thirty men interviewed had at least one, and sometimes several, episodes of venereal disease as adolescents and young adults. There was a lot of competition among classmates for girls. Many students had an ambivalent attitude toward venereal disease. While some considered it the inevitable conqueror's "battle scar," others read it as a sign of carelessness, a failure to attract the right "class" of girls. A lack of discrimination had led them to choose "finished" girls, who were obvious sources of infection. At school, especially in their last year, many boys had local girlfriends who lived in nearby villages and who were either attending primary school or who had "dropped out" at grade seven or much earlier.[14]

Religious Education

One of the major themes of *Christian Living Today* (CLT, 1975), the senior religious education syllabus followed at St. Antony's was "Man and Woman." Designed to be acceptable to a range of Christian churches, the syllabus, taught throughout Zambia, was developed by a committee of Catholics and Protestants from Kenya, Malawi, Tanzania, Uganda, and Zambia for use in secondary schools in these countries. The emphasis was on *"education for life"* (1975: 1), the starting point being *"the student's own experience"* (ibid., italics in the original). Many former students took the course, though few of them referred to it directly in our conversations around the end of their school careers. An appendix on human sexuality described in ideal terms "Stages of Human Sexual Development" and "Aspects of Personality Development in Boys and Girls." Though not explicitly acknowledged, in the latter section, the influence of a rather benign interpretation of Freudian psychology is evident, especially, for example, in the discussion of the father-son relationship:

> At about 4, 5 and 6 the boy wants not only to receive love, but also to give it, especially to his mother. To some degree he becomes jealous of his father, who shares the mother's affection. In order to win affection from his mother, he tries to act like his father. This is the first time he begins to identify himself as a male person. His love of his mother leads to a loving imitation of his father.... (1975: 132)

There is no suggestion here of the fear of the father that most former students recalled. Again, regarding the ages between six and nine, and contrary to the childhood play experiences recalled by the men, the syllabus notes that "boys and girls at this age are not interested in their sexual differences" (ibid.). The term birth control was used as a synonym for planned parenthood. There was no mention of condoms. The syllabus did not set out only Catholic teaching that forbade anything other than abstinence and the rhythm method in marriage. Rather the importance of having sufficient requirements to bring up children in an adequate manner was highlighted.

Pregnancies

A third of the former students interviewed fathered children, or caused pregnancies, while they were primary or secondary school students. As the boys grew older, most of them thought that their parents were aware of their sexual exploits. The veil of silence between a teenager and his parents was torn when a girl's family accused a boy of causing her pregnancy. The boy's family would usually offer to pay "damages" for the pregnancy and sometimes give promises of marriage, which were rarely, if ever, kept once the boy had finished school. Boys' parents tried to prevent these cases being drawn to the attention of the school authorities who, in theory, were obliged to report them to the Ministry of Education. In the 1980s the penalty was expulsion. Mwanakatwe, the first minister of education, had stressed the need for sexual discipline. Singling out girls for particular rebuke, he highlighted "the intolerable misconduct" (Mwanakatwe 1968: 236) of pregnant schoolgirls and endorsed the UNIP government's hard-line policy of expelling the girls and the boys who were responsible for such exploits. He reminded readers: "In tribal society an unmarried girl who became pregnant was regarded as a social outcast; indeed under Zulu law the sanction against parties responsible for illegitimate pregnancies was death" (ibid.). He argued against the readmission of schoolgirls after the delivery of their babies, expressing the view that their readmission "would degrade educational institutions."[15]

At fifteen, in grade seven, Enoch learnt that he had made his girlfriend pregnant. He had built his own hut in the village and she had slept with him. He had not realized that at his age he could cause a pregnancy. He thought only "big people" [adults] could produce children. When the case was brought before the village headman, Enoch denied paternity even though he was convinced that he was responsible. He explained to me: "It was something I did unknowingly. We had been sleeping together and I had released into her most nights." He was afraid of losing his chance of secondary education. The girl had stopped school some years earlier in grade three. After her death, and his marriage, Enoch took the child to live with him.

Promise's build and athletic skill attracted many girls and he had several sexual partners in the later stages of his primary education. It did not occur to him to use condoms. He formed a particularly close relationship with a grade-six girl. (She has since died.) In grade seven Promise, at the age of fourteen, discovered she was pregnant. She told him he was responsible. Unsure whether he was "rescued by chance," Promise explained: "Fortunately there was a miscarriage. Well, I don't know whether she aborted or whether it was a miscarriage. It was fortunate because I was still young. What could I do? Anyway we both qualified for grade eight." The girl's family sued Promise. He described the contrasting reactions of his parents. His father, he recalled, "didn't bother much" and paid one of his cattle in compensation. His mother, however, was furious that he had put his education at risk.

In the 1980s interviews, young men, with few exceptions, maintained that premarital sex was "normal." In a student initiation that students called "mockery," grade eight newcomers to St. Antony's had to prove their manhood and thereby their right to belong in tales of sexual experience given in a speech at night in the dormitories. (See Simpson 2003: 128–134.) Sex was to be enjoyed. Most young men spoke of "playing sex"—a direct translation from local languages such as the Bemba verb *ukukwangala*, which means "to play."[16] Yet, while sex before marriage was to be enjoyed, for many it was still "against the Bible," "like stealing" and therefore "a sin." Some expected God to punish them. While they greatly appreciated the education offered by the Catholic Brothers, who vowed to live a celibate life and who were dedicated to the Virgin Mary, they were puzzled by the expressions of masculinity that the missionaries embodied. Richards observed that Bemba attitudes revealed that they considered sexual intercourse as "necessary to normal wellbeing, and a pleasure to which all are entitled" (1969: 15). Dover (2005) describes similar ideas in the lower Zambezi valley about the importance of regular sexual intercourse for health and wellbeing. Richards commented of the Bemba people, "Chastity in the sense of complete abstinence is not a recognized ideal at any stage of life, whether before or after marriage, and the bulk of pagan

Natives consider the prenuptial chastity demanded by the missionary as an almost fantastic conception—to judge from some of their comments—and the practice of celibacy as incredible" (1969: 15). (See also Hinfelaar 1994.)

Many students expressed their skepticism that Catholic missionaries did indeed live according to their declared ideal. A celibate person could not, in their view, ever be truly happy. First there was the need to find relief from the sexual tension a "normal" person must feel. Beyond that, sexual activity was a way of keeping healthy. Using the scientific language of school, they explained that their own early sexual activity was largely driven by the desire to experiment and gain the experience necessary for adult life and marriage. They feared that their wives might find them wanting in their sexual performance.[17] They frequently remarked in their late teens, "You can't expect a virgin wife when you marry."[18]

Masturbation

Competitive masturbation revealed how the forceful ejaculation of sperm became for most young men the measure of the "real man." Many boys had discovered masturbation entirely on their own, while others had been taught by male peers. Enoch told me he had learnt from a friend, though he did not enjoy it. A male friend had also taught Peter to masturbate, but he recalled that he found the experience boring and he was "not excited enough" to continue the practice. Elders warned boys that masturbation would lead to impotence and some boys agreed.[19] Like attitudes to same-sex sex, the general opinion was that masturbation could not provide much pleasure. Dominic, at forty, spoke of his personal experience: "Well, I have masturbated but the way I look at it, well, masturbating—it's not very satisfying. It's something that you imagine and then you do it but it is not very satisfying."

Student views on masturbation ranged from condemnation to qualified tolerance. Some young men expressed opprobrium, usually on religious grounds, saying that it was "abnormal." An excessive interest in self-masturbation was thought by some to lead to, or be an indication of, homosexuality. They said such practices were "against the Bible," though no one mentioned Onan,[20] and besides masturbation entailed wasting semen and creating matter out of place.[21] Hambayi, at twenty a member of the Seventh Day Adventist Church, spoke of his strong disapproval, suspecting that anyone living without regular sexual intercourse, and here he included the Catholic missionaries, would seek relief in masturbation and homosexual activity:

> Nowhere is it written that you should not marry. God has given us the green light. He wants us to produce. Now, if someone says, "Me, I'm not going to marry," why? No, that one, I don't see it to be a normal way of living, not the way we are created as human beings, as men. There is that sexual desire, unless you are sick. Now, if you are not sick, what do you do? That's why people resort to malpractices such as, excuse me, it's not an insult, masturbation, even homosexuality.[22] I mean these things are not supposed to be there. A woman is supposed to be used. Why should you do it on your own? I mean you are destroying now. Instead of building something, you are wasting.

Many students, among them Kangwa, Henry, and Paul—who all identified themselves as Catholics—saw nothing wrong with masturbation, though they maintained that they did not find it "exciting." Most boys thought that regular masturbation helped to enlarge and strengthen the penis—a desirable outcome, even if it entailed loss of semen and hence, in their understanding, potency. Mutual masturbation was not mentioned in the religious education syllabus. Self-masturbation was dealt with briefly and sympathetically, where it was recognized: "Occasional masturbation can be a normal part of adolescent self-discovery" (CLT 1975: 132).[23]

In general, young men had thought of masturbation simply as a means of relief from the buildup of pressure caused by the absence of regular sex, though they spoke also of the need for a degree of self-control. Frequency was an issue. Once or twice a month, for some, was considered reasonable; more frequent than that was thought to lead either to a disinterest in women and or an inability to satisfy them, often because of premature ejaculation. Paul, at nineteen, commented, "Even in the religious view it is accepted as normal; it is not harmful. If it is erring, it is erring on the safe side; it is better than fornication." The general attitude among senior students was that there was little need to masturbate at boarding school as one could always find a girl, either in the surrounding villages or during visits to the nearby town. However, it was recognized that some young men were too shy, lacking the "courage" and facility with persuasive words required to "hook" a girl. Boys who were not known to engage in sex with local girls, but who were suspected of finding "relief" in masturbation, were mocked.

Several men recalled masturbating with age-mates in demonstrations of the achievement of manhood—that is, a large penis and the ability to ejaculate semen speedily and forcefully.[24] Promise described his own experience of masturbation from the age of ten or eleven years of age, over a period of more than two years, involving not only age-mates but considerably older boys—indeed, young men who took an active role in masturbating him. In Promise's account, as in those of others, the association between physical strength, sexual strength, and social capital is clear. Herd boys were paired to fight according to what were judged to be their relative sexual potency, as Promise explained:

> It used to be very interesting. The older boys used to make us fight. Fight! Maybe, they could first of all start with animals. First the animals fight—bulls from different kraals. Then later we make a ring. We start fighting. First they see if you produce sperms or not. You see they were trying to find the right person to fight with. If you do not produce sperms, the two of you fight. If you produce sperms, the two of you, then you fight. These bigger boys, well, some of them were young men, some even twenty years old, we used to move with them when we were herding, well, they were forcing us to masturbate. Some of those bigger boys, they were at school with us. Others had already stopped. They were just herdsmen. At times, they would masturbate us, especially when you were just brought in the group at the beginning, but also later; they could come and start masturbating you. I really don't know why they would do that. Well, sometimes they could just come there. Maybe you are masturbating, but maybe you are doing it slowly. At times they wanted to find out who produced sperms fast, who released sperms faster than the others. You start, "On your marks, get set, go!" You all start masturbating. Then they would find out who releases faster. So sometimes they would masturbate you. Now being faster—ah, you are praised, you are praised, "He's a man! He's a man! Yeah! He's the fastest! He's a man!" So you see speed was important. One, the speed, two, the pressure at which the stuff was produced, that is the distance when you are standing. Yes, these are the two things. They were telling us to do it, trying to find out our manhood. Whenever we met, we were asked to masturbate. And mostly what attracted these bigger boys was the power, the power—that is the strength at which the sperms were released. You see, there were those other sperms which were just released. I mean they could come out just like water. But then there were those sperms, which were released with strength—shooting up, yes. At times you could do it lying, at times standing. Yes. They would be looking at you, judging who was stronger by judging how far the sperms were going. If you were the best they would shout, "You are a man! You are a man!" (Laughing.)

Promise did not remember feeling shy when masturbating with other boys or being masturbated by them, as he did when he first had penetrative sex with a girl. Rather he recalled the pleasure he felt in being praised by other boys when he was found to be the "best" in the production of semen. He delighted in being recognized as "the boss" among his age-mates, who had to obey his orders and perform the tasks he formerly had to perform, such as going in search of a stray animal. He enjoyed the sexual pleasure, the sense of relief, but he did not consider this activity as in any way out-of-the-ordinary. It was, he explained, "just something that used to happen—a form of leisure—just part of us."

In adult life, most former students would speak of self-masturbation as a practice understandable in children and adolescents, though unsuitable for mature men, indeed rather shameful. Some reported asking their wives, or other sexual partners, to masturbate them as a substitute form of "relief" because of taboos against intercourse during menstruation. (See chapter 6.) Suggestions that mutual masturbation as an alternative for penetrative sex might be a possible strategy for avoiding HIV/AIDS risk were dismissed as completely untenable. Sexually active, schoolgoing teenagers in Lusaka have been reported to hold a similar view. (See Feldman et al. 1997.)

Conclusion

Much of the playfulness that surrounded early sexual experimentation would soon be lost in the shadow of AIDS. Children did their best to imitate adults. In sexual play they tried to behave like "normal," "healthy" people. Boys, left, in the main, to work out things for themselves, strove to attain the "manly" position of command, to take the "active" role, despite their fear of failure. However, their sexual inexperience often made them the pupils of experienced, usually older, girls. In the course of the lifecycle, with the transformation at marriage of girlfriends into wives, young women would lose much of the sexual freedom they had enjoyed in childhood and adolescence. Boys increasingly felt the pressure, especially from peers, to behave in a manly fashion, to demonstrate their competence at sexual conquest and strength in their performance of sexual intercourse. They sought *muti* to masculinize their bodies; they competed in urinating and masturbating competitions in their claim for acceptance among fellow boys. A reputation for successful performances earned them kudos among peers. Despite reports that the majority of Zambian secondary school students disapprove of premarital sex (see Mufune et al. 1993), their disapproval does not appear to be a realistic indication of their day-to-day lives (see Warenius et al. [2007]). Yet secondary school students in Zambia continue to lack adequate information about human reproduction and sexual health. The picture offered here of male adolescent sexual experience twenty or thirty years ago is mirrored by recent studies of boys in Zambia. Dählback et al. (2003: 57), for example, report that the primary reason given by adolescent boys in Zambia for starting sexual activity at an early age is peer pressure. Boys in Lusaka and the Copperbelt perceive sexuality and fertility as the core of manhood (ibid. 55). Koster-Oyekan reports, in her study of abortion in Zambia's Western Province, that 58 percent of the secondary school girls from grades ten to twelve, surveyed or interviewed, reported having had sex (1998: 1306). She notes estimates of high numbers of secondary school girls in the country dropping out of school because of pregnancy, thereby highlighting once more the need for adolescent health provision.

At St. Antony's, biology classes and religious education lessons furnished some information about sexuality. Boys might describe premarital sexual intercourse as a "sin," but this did not deter them. However, they set moral parameters. "Moderate" sexual activity was condoned, but in the view of the majority masturbating too frequently or using condoms indicated excess that needed to be curbed. Indeed, even when available, condoms were, and remained, extremely unpopular. They might be used early in a relationship. But, instead of being perceived as barriers to infection, they were rejected as obstacles to pleasure, speed of ejaculation, intimacy, and trust. The attitudes of these students at St. Antony's regarding condom use are in line with those reported of young men elsewhere. Flood (2003), for example, offers striking similarities with the views of young heterosexual Australian men, particularly with regard to complaints of loss of penile sensation, privileging trust, and developing intimacy as explanations for nonuse. For problems associated with condom use among migrant workers in Zambia, see Bond and Dover (1997). For estimates of condom use on the Zambian Copperbelt, see Buvé et al. (2001).

Though from a wide range of socioeconomic backgrounds, as members of an elite-in-the-making, St. Antony's students imagined themselves as having the pick both of girls they considered to be of their own class and of poorer and younger girls from the nearby primary school and villages. They might promise the latter marriage if a pregnancy case was brought against them, but none of these promises were kept. Indeed, most young men's strategy was to deny paternity.

Apart from such moments, silence reigned between children and parents on sexual matters even when, perhaps especially when, young boys experienced what they would later identify as sexual abuse.

After school their life courses would follow different trajectories. Further education, type of employment and unemployment, economic power, foreign travel for work, church affiliation, and various personal attributes, all would contribute to where they situated themselves—or found themselves situated—in relation to local hegemonic notions of masculinity. Young men in the 1980s had said that they were always conscious of the need to "carry convincing stories back to school" after the holidays, though some students, like Paul, recalled that they were often able to concoct some story simply from listening to others telling of their sexual escapades. In later life, despite some marriages that clearly challenged the prevailing gender order, my fieldwork reveals that many men among this group remained under the sway of the often unspoken contest with other men to prove their virility. Education, especially that of Catholic missionaries, would prove no protection as they strove to express their sexuality and to convince themselves and others of their manliness. They continued to feel the pressure of their peers. Despite their growing awareness of the terrible toll that the AIDS pandemic exacted, they engaged in unprotected sex with multiple partners, thereby increasing the risks of becoming infected and infecting others with HIV.

4

Sexual Lives after School

At school, many students intended to marry only when they were in a position to provide for a wife and children. Where a student was the only member of his family to progress as far as grade twelve, and especially if he expected to gain a university degree, he anticipated having to provide for younger siblings' upkeep and education. He also imagined that he would be required to give financial support to his parents and, on occasion, to various members of his and his wife's family. Students recognized "real" manliness entailed becoming the "breadwinner." The majority, expecting to proceed to tertiary education, anticipated that marriage would be postponed at least until around the age of thirty. Besides, in their late teens and early twenties, they considered themselves to be too immature for marriage, "still excited," "too unstable." An extended school career seemed to have persuaded them of their immaturity, so unlike their age-mates who had "failed" to get into secondary school and who by their early twenties were often married, especially those who lived in rural areas.[1]

While students insisted they would not allow their parents to choose a wife for them, few thought they could go ahead with a marriage that their parents disapproved of. What the young men did not anticipate, though it became quite common, was that they would provide financial support for their wives-to-be, in some instances, for a number of years prior to marriage, setting up a relationship of dependence. Receiving such support during school or college training meant for a woman the acceptance of a sexual relationship. Without exception, marriage was tied to the idea of producing children as much for the men as for the women. In general, the young men expected to have a smaller number of children than their parents' generation, citing the difficult economic circumstances facing Zambia in the 1980s and the greater financial demands of town- as opposed to village life.[2] Economic conditions also figured in students' rejection of polygamy, though many expressed the fear that jealous co-wives might make them sick with love potions or even try to poison them. Several students, like Promise and Hambayi, had polygamous fathers. Promise did not entirely rule out the possibility of becoming a polygamist in later life. His father brought a succession of women into the home, each of whom Promise had been required to acknowledge as his stepmother, after his parents' divorce.[3] Hambayi's mother was the first of his father's three wives. For many years there were only two. Hambayi recalled a happy childhood in which his two mothers got on well and jointly cared for his father's thirteen children. Indeed it was his father's co-wife who had cared for him in infancy and even given him his name. From his observation of his father's married life, Hambayi commented, "The man in our tradition capitalizes. The husband receives 'double services,' his bath water is warmed by one or another wife and his food is often prepared by the two of them." However, Hambayi recalled that when his father introduced a third, much younger wife, his mother became sad and withdrawn as she no longer attracted a major share of her husband's attention.

My Future Wife

In the essays the students had written for me in senior secondary school in the 1980s on the topic of "My Future Wife," certain common themes emerged. Apart from the need for her to be beautiful, that is "light-brown in complexion" and, if possible, to have "a triangular nose, like a European," most students stressed that she must be "obedient." She should be sufficiently educated to be able to contribute to household finances. The general opinion was that she should have at least completed grade twelve, though some said grade nine or ten would be sufficient. This would guarantee that she would be able to express herself properly and know how to deal with others. However, no student wanted a wife whose level of education surpassed his. Most stressed that their wives should value "African tradition," and indeed be African; a wife should be respectful to her husband and to visitors, readily welcoming members of the man's family when they came to stay. She should not resent the financial help her husband might give them. While most students said that ethnic group membership would not be an important factor, they almost all insisted that she would have to be a Christian. Many worried about having a troublesome or quarrelsome wife.

In our conversations at the end of their schooldays, the young men invariably imagined the process as one where *they* would choose a partner, never for a moment imagining that they might be the ones chosen. Several of them pointed to local languages that used the active voice of the verb to marry for the man and the passive voice for the woman.[4] When it came to choosing a wife, a young woman's character would count more than her looks. The general opinion was that ideally a wife should be between five and ten years younger than her husband because, students explained, once women started to have children they lost their looks and aged much more quickly than men. Most stressed they desired a partner who would provide care and companionship, someone who would be "understanding." Chimbala, who was to marry at twenty-eight and to die of AIDS in his mid-thirties, leaving a wife and three children, exemplified this desire when he was nineteen:

> I think I will get married between thirty and thirty-five. The woman should first of all be kind. She should be understanding and forgiving. She should be younger because, as they say, if we are the same age, the woman will grow old faster than me. She should be at least good-looking and well built.[5] Tribe doesn't matter but she should have at least some education and be able to work and earn some money. In that way we can help one another.

For Hambayi, at twenty, the woman's character and background would be the deciding factors. These would only be discovered by investigating the woman's family. His decision to marry would be based on love and not on tribe or religion. As far as education was concerned, it would depend on whether he chose to live in town or in his village: "At home [in his village] education is not really valued there because there is nothing to write. All you have got to do is farming and, well, for women at least; they don't need education for farming."

At twenty, Kangwa had anticipated that he would marry around the age of twenty-five. He had a clear picture of his future wife and, like *some* of his contemporaries, he offered me a rather romantic picture:

> She's got to be understanding and kind. Above all she must love me. She mustn't love me because of what I have or the position that I hold because I believe there is that natural love. There is love that comes without reason. Maybe when I ask her, "Why do you love me?" she won't even be able to answer.... She would have to have a certain level of education; a minimum would be grade ten.

Kangwa expected to have a number of sexual partners between the end of his schooldays and marriage and wondered how his wife would compare to them: "I believe I might not get the kind of excitement from my wife that I get from a mere girlfriend. Now, when I don't get that experience, that excitement, from my wife, well, I will judge my wife's coolness and this will cause problems." Chimbala too revealed his anxiety on this score: "By the time I marry I expect to have had a lot of sexual experience. But the one I marry will probably also have had a lot of partners. It bothers me. She might not be faithful. She might make comparisons and I might feel I wasn't as good at love-making as the others she has known."

At twenty, Mutinta said he thought it would be at least ten years before he would feel "mature enough, settled economically, socially and emotionally." He commented, "When you are mature, that's when you can take on the responsibilities of life." Mutinta felt he had yet to experience "falling in love" with a girl. Beyond her being beautiful, his wife could be "anyone who is head over heels in love with me."

Kabwe, the sixth-born of fourteen children, thought a good age to marry would be after twenty-five. At twenty, he considered the purpose of marriage was "childbearing" and that premarital sex was important to ensure that the couple were sexually compatible. Like a number of others he hoped to find a partner with whom he would be able to enjoy a companionable marriage. By the end of secondary school Kabwe, who was to die from AIDS in his late twenties, had had four sexual partners since his first "proper" sex at seventeen. He exemplified the common acceptance among students that they would face a range of expectations from relatives for material support:

> I will marry when I can live nicely and when I can take care of my young brothers. I can think of marriage at a time when I am able to help others. My ideal partner would be someone who could help me.... She should also be someone who is not selfish, someone who would not refuse to keep my relatives. I come from a big family and my parents are aging. The young ones will need someone to look after them—I will have to keep them. It would be difficult if I married someone who wouldn't like to keep my young brothers and sisters at home. Such things would drive me to divorce. On the other hand, I would also want to look after her relatives. She would have to have some education. I can't see someone who is illiterate being able to help me.

Paul had had no intention of marrying before the age of twenty-five. In fact he did not marry until he was twenty-eight. At eighteen, he had abandoned what he considered the childish notion that the most important thing was that his wife should be beautiful. For him, the character of his future wife was the key; she would have to be someone who would make a good mother for his children. Falling in love would not create a sound foundation for a marriage. Eighteen-year-old Henry had expected to marry in his early thirties after completing university and establishing himself in his chosen career. He did not think that tribe, nationality, or religion would play a part in his choice of wife:

> She should be a person who is very understanding. She should accept my way of life. We should know each other very well and for some time before we marry. She should be good-looking. She should have a substantial education—perhaps be a university graduate—but not above my own qualifications because such girls might boast about their bigger salary. They might use their greater salary or their education as a weapon against me in a quarrel, for example.

Young men dreamed of being in command in their marriage, yet their fervent hope was that they would find a supportive and caring wife. Little did they know the degree to which older women would instruct their future wives how to care for them and to practice patience and tolerance. Mission education and the desire to secure economic independence meant that they had many years in which to "experiment" with potential partners, though they would remain anxious about their ability to give and receive sexual satisfaction. For some men, the dream of marriage and family would be short-lived, as within years of starting a family they would be dead from what was assumed to be AIDS. For many, marital relationships would come to be marked by distrust.

Becoming "Loose"

In the mid- and late 1980s most of the young men interviewed, like their fellow students at St. Antony's, were convinced that HIV/AIDS that they were just beginning to hear about was no threat to them. Their immediate fears concerned pregnancies and venereal diseases. Almost without exception, they did not consider life without sex viable. The majority continued to "chance" and have "live" sex, that is, intercourse without a condom. Numbers of premarital sexual partners varied; some men spoke of three or four, some of twenty, thirty, or sixty. Others said they were unable to give an accurate estimate, a common phrase being "quite a queue." Several had very few partners and there was the exceptional case of Peter, who maintained that he delayed sexual intercourse until marriage.

For many, immediately after school there was a marked increase in the number of sexual partners. Their first task was to find paid employment. Few could afford to sit at home, waiting for their exam results. However, finding a job, without contacts among family, friends, or fellow church members was extremely difficult. The very limited job market was annually swamped with grade nine and grade twelve school-leavers. Many found temporary employment as "untrained teachers." The Ministry of Education employed those who had completed grade twelve to teach in primary schools. School-leavers were often posted to remote rural schools where it was difficult to attract and retain trained teachers.[6] Former students enjoyed teaching, though they were usually poorly housed and went for months without pay. They spoke about their newfound sense of freedom, living away from home and for the first time enjoying some measure of financial independence. In retrospect, with regard to their sexual activities, many described themselves as becoming "loose" and "rough." Some had sex with their female primary school pupils, but most of them had encounters with single and married women of their own age and older. In remote rural areas, an unmarried secondary school-leaver was a highly eligible bachelor. Enoch estimated that during his two years as an untrained teacher at a rural school he had had about twenty sexual partners. He claimed that many unmarried women signaled to him that they were interested in a sexual relationship, in his view, because they were eager for marriage. Despite causing his girlfriend's pregnancy at primary school, Enoch did not use condoms. Promise taught at two rural primary schools. He too described this as a time when he became "loose." Within two years he had a total of seven sexual relationships and fathered two children with two women. In his second posting, Promise said he "proposed love" to his headmaster's young teenage daughter. From his account, it is clear that he coerced her. He explained, "I must say I tried to force that relationship. I just forced her. She was young. She was refusing. I wouldn't say it was a successful relationship with her; I released [ejaculated] outside." Her father ensured that he did not get any further untrained teaching posts.

Former students tried other ways of making a living. Maxwell, the fifth-born in a family of eight children, returned to live with his mother in an urban compound where he set up a small tavern. For three years business was good, but then a series of robberies rendered him bankrupt. He went to work as a casual laborer on building sites around the city. Managing to save a little money, he bought secondhand clothes that his father took to his home village in Southern Province to exchange for maize which Maxwell then sold back in Lusaka. Within a short time he had tripled his initial investment and he ploughed his profits into buying and selling stationery. This too went well for a time and he decided to go to Botswana and Zimbabwe and engage in cross-border trade, first cosmetics and paint and later gemstones and mobile phones. His mother also traveled regularly by bus to Zimbabwe, bringing back blankets and shoes to sell. She had managed to raise enough money to buy a sewing machine and was now making clothes for sale. In 2002, thin and looking permanently exhausted, Maxwell was struggling to make ends meet. Customers in Zambia took a long time to pay for the goods they agreed to buy. A down payment was promptly given when the goods were delivered, but collecting the balance would take months and involve repeated visits to workplaces and homes. Maxwell spent most days walking around the city trying to collect what he was owed and making contacts that might provide a financial return. He recalled having sex with two girls while at primary school and with five while at secondary school. Describing himself as "a decent guy," he explained that, unlike some of his contemporaries, he had "really behaved" after leaving school. Between school and getting married at the age of twenty-eight, he had had sex with "only four women," apart from his fiancée, though one of the relationships had continued while she was away following a course of studies that he was paying for. He had also once paid for sex, though he stressed that it was his friend's idea: "I wasn't in the mood but my friend persuaded me, two of us and two women. We paid twenty thousand for each girl for a few hours. I was forced into it. The girl was loose. She convinced me."

Darius had sex with several women while he was involved in cross-border trade. Having fathered two children soon after leaving school, he had tried always to use condoms in his sexual encounters. In the early 1990s he met a teenage schoolgirl: "She told me she was a virgin and I believed [her]. Then I started having sex without a condom again. We promised each other marriage up to the time she disappointed [me]. I was keen to marry her. I really wanted to have a child with her but she kept aborting." His girlfriend had three abortions in all, her first at seventeen during her secondary education, in Darius's opinion, because she was afraid of her parents' reaction should they discover that she was pregnant. He wanted to have a child with her and to be socially recognized as the father of the child. He thought that a child would strengthen their relationship. After she finished school, again without her parents' knowledge, they started living together but another abortion followed. Angry, Darius started a concurrent relationship with another young woman, a grade eleven student at a local secondary school. He planned to marry her. His desire for intimacy and pleasure together with his wish to father a child led Darius to forego condoms, once he had "studied" her and decided that she was not "mischievous," that is, was not having sex with anyone else. She gave birth to a son while she was still living at her parents' home. However, her family's opposition prevented him from seeing her or their child. Darius then began a relationship with another young woman, a grade twelve student. The relationship continued after his marriage. He did not use condoms, he explained, "out of excitement." He recalled that they would both drink heavily and go to bed drunk. He had persuaded her to take contraceptive pills in order not to put her education in jeopardy. Nevertheless, she became pregnant. He provided money for her requirements and the baby's needs. She subsequently married another man who was persuaded by her into believing that the child was his. However, she continued her sexual relationship with Darius when opportunities arose. Darius was unsure how long she had been having a relationship with both men. He had wanted a child, but he reconciled himself to the fact that she had chosen somebody else to be responsible for what, in retrospect, he called his "mistake."

Very soon after leaving school, Malama started a sexual relationship with a girl who within a few months became pregnant. His parents, who had never spoken to him about sex, expressed their displeasure. He recalled their admonition: "My parents said, 'You see, you should not have sex before you marry! It is bad and in God's eyes it is a sin. And you do not know. This might even lead you to marrying someone when you don't want to, or plan to.'" After the birth of the baby, Malama lost contact with the girl. He heard that she subsequently married a man in a village not far from her own.

After school Sampa tried various jobs, before becoming a company salesman. Access to a vehicle and money gave him opportunities for sexual encounters. He found many women, single and married, ready to have sexual intercourse with him in exchange for beer and gifts, some of them samples of his company's products. When a woman was reluctant, he explained he would "become impatient and buy her with presents." In the early 1990s Sampa went to a neighboring country to attend a six-month course. The women he encountered there were, he explained, quite unlike the majority of Zambian women he had known. "A true Zambian woman cannot tell you to put on a condom!" he told me, unlike these women who were "very strict" about condoms. Shortly after his return to Zambia, Sampa lost his job. Back at his home in the compound he started to run a shebeen. His reported command over women because of their desire for, or addiction to, beer had echoes of his *modus operandi* at school, when as "teacher," he had sexual access to schoolgirls. He later reflected, in the light of the deaths of family and friends from AIDS:

> With so many women ready to have sex with you in return for beer, you risked your life. The women brought themselves. There was no forcing on my part. I would just say, "No, you, at the end of the day, I am with you." You talk, you talk, you are on top of her. I can't remember the exact number but probably around forty or fifty different women. Sometimes I used condoms but mostly I didn't. If a woman asked for a condom, it meant the woman was clean. So I didn't use one. Then again, you look at a girl and think, "No, this one, she can't have a disease. She looks like a clean lady. Let me go direct!"

Sampa again suffered from sexually transmitted infections, this time "three-in-one," gonorrhea, syphilis, and *bolabola* (*lymphogranuloma inguinale*). He attended a clinic for treatment. As more and more friends succumbed to the ravages of AIDS, Sampa said he became more conscious of the risks he was taking. For a short while he engaged in cross-border trade. He traveled with his mother both to assist her and to have her as a form of protection against the attractions of the women traders he encountered. He found this "less risky" and said he had sex with "only three women" in this period. Considering these "business women" to be the most likely carriers of sexually transmitted infections, and especially the HIV virus, he used condoms at all times with them.

At University

About half of the men interviewed were graduates from the University of Zambia. Most had gone to university a year after they had completed secondary school, though two had completed a degree as in-service teachers. University undergraduates in the 1980s received generous bursaries that at times exceeded what some would earn when they qualified and started working. In the Zambian context, they were generally perceived to be very privileged people. At the

University of Zambia, competition for girls was particularly acute. In the mid-1980s, Dominic felt great peer pressure both to engage in bouts of beer drinking and to have a girlfriend in a student culture where, he explained, "there was a tradition of a lot of sex. If you didn't have a girlfriend, you felt there must be something wrong with you." Having a girlfriend was, he emphasized, a way of "showing others that you were a man." He found that a man without a girlfriend was ostracized. Every year of his university course Dominic had at least one girlfriend, with whom he regularly had unprotected sex. Like his fellow graduates, he noted there was little talk about the risk of contracting the HIV virus.

As an undergraduate, Simon lived in the oldest student accommodation on campus that students had named "The Ruins." Situated furthermost away from the women students' hostels, it was also called "Monks"—a place where "monks" lived. In student parlance, "monks" were the men who did not have any regular girlfriends, whereas "mojos" were those who did. Simon felt the pressure to be seen to have a girlfriend. But his sexual experience was, he considered, very limited—having had sex with only three girls since his first sexual intercourse at the age of seventeen. He felt extremely shy. He wanted to approach girls but he did not know how to begin. No one had taught him. The skill of successfully approaching a woman for sex was expected to come naturally for a man. Though at university he found making friends with girls easy, he did not know how to start a sexual relationship with them. In retrospect he thought his biggest fear through his teenage years and in his twenties had been rejection. Besides, he was ambitious to do well in his chosen career and was not eager for distractions. Fellow students might call him a "monk," but his determination to succeed enabled him to ignore their taunts, especially as he knew that many first-year students were excluded from the university because they failed to qualify for the second year. He was determined not to be one of them. Besides, he knew it was difficult for first-year males to "hook" female undergraduates. While female undergraduates did not easily conform to young men's expectations of subservience, many were ready to engage in sexual relationships with senior students, academic members of staff, and older wealthy men. Simon observed, "When you are in the university in your first year, everyone considers you to be—as a man—you are crap." Nevertheless, most students were successful in "hooking" a girl in their first year, though they may not have exclusive sexual access to her. Mutinta's shyness and introversion persisted into adult life. However, his sporting skills at university attracted a number of girls. In his first year a second-year woman student approached him. He recollected, "The girl negotiated me! She was already experienced in these things." After that relationship ended, Mutinta recalled a number of "only irrelevant encounters—not proper relationships." He always used condoms at university, not because of AIDS, he explained, but to prevent pregnancies. He did not feel ready for any permanent commitment that he feared would be required of him, should he father a child.

In general there was greater reported use of condoms among university students than among their school contemporaries; though, according to former students, this was on *their* initiative and not at women's insistence, and was usually discontinued as a relationship developed. Edmund had several sexual partners at university. Exceptionally, after school, the condom became a must, he claimed, regardless of how much beer he had drunk. Unlike most of his friends, who complained about loss of sensation, he argued that consistent condom use was not difficult. At forty and recently married, he commented, "How do you tell that it is sweet before you enter? I think it is all in the mind." Losing four brothers and other relatives and friends to what was assumed to be AIDS strengthened his resolve never to have unprotected sex outside marriage. Besides, he had ambition, to get promotion at work, and one day to have a family. His job after university gave him access to an unlimited supply of free condoms. He insisted on always using them, though some of his girlfriends tried to dissuade him. In his view they wanted to build trust by having unprotected sex. He tactfully stressed that he was protecting his partner as much as himself by refusing to engage in unprotected sex. In his first year Henry also managed to have a girlfriend, with whom he enjoyed regular sex though the relationship ended in tragic circumstances. In the second year he had another girlfriend, but at the end of her first year she dropped out of university and began paid employment. She subsequently terminated their relationship, in Henry's view, because he was not earning money and so was unable to match her income or provide for her. He did not always use condoms and caused one pregnancy that was terminated. His schoolboy fears had come true.

Paul recalled the popularity of discos and nightclubs during his time at university. He would regularly visit discos with fellow undergraduates. His older brother, Robert, also took him drinking at the most popular nightclubs in Lusaka. At one nightspot Paul could make out the figures of numerous couples copulating on sheets of cardboard spread out by security guards in the grounds of the club. He thought they were "out of their minds." Paul later counted the numerous "stars," the young men and women who made such an impression there, who had been swept away, most of them—like Robert—dead from AIDS. One of Paul's brothers-in-law, who was also later to die from AIDS, was a heavy beer drinker. He would take Paul out drinking for the whole night, chiding him about his apparent lack of interest in women and boasting of his own youthful sexual exploits, Paul recalled:

> Can you imagine? Even though he was my brother-in-law, he would have the courage to say, "Ah, me, when I was your age—I was 'Bazooka.' A bazooka! That was what I was called. All those girls knew me!" You know, as if to say to me, why are you wasting your talents, wasting your time? Why? You know, you should be busy gunning for all these ladies around! Something like that.

Paul was embarrassed rather than inspired by such exhortations. His determination to avoid intercourse was strengthened at the end of his first year of university when he shared a room in "The Ruins" with a Born Again Christian who for a while had "backslid." They prayed and studied the Bible together; this renewed Paul's determination to avoid sexual intercourse. He started praying at a Pentecostal church and also with other Born Again students on campus, but some of them, he explained "went into sin of a sexual nature and failed to repent." Paul became disillusioned and stopped attending. It would be five years before he would again seek a church where he might pray with others.

Throughout the 1980s and 1990s, there were several bars near the university campus where students paid for sex, usually standing against the back wall of the building. In 2002 sex remained available at such bars at the cost of 5,000 kwacha a round with a condom. Many women insisted on a condom, though for 30,000 kwacha some women were prepared to have unprotected sex.

Getting Married

Most former students' first marriage took place when they were between the ages of twenty-five and thirty. Typically, brides were some years younger, at times by as much as ten years, though there were some instances of age-mates marrying. Several women were still in secondary school when the relationships began. While a man's decision to marry depended on economic circumstances, men explained to me that increasing awareness of HIV/AIDS played an important part. With more and more people they knew dying from what was assumed to be AIDS, many of the men interviewed concluded that they would be safer if they married. In addition to the status and comforts that a wife would bring, several former students reasoned that as married men they would have sex readily available, and so would not be driven to seek relief and satisfaction with whomsoever it could be found. Darius, who married at twenty-five, explained, "I am scared of AIDS. If anything that is what has made me settle with my current wife. That is why I wouldn't move from her to another lady." He simply set up home with his partner who was, atypically among his contemporaries' wives, four years older than he. Some of his family accepted the marriage, while others considered her too old for him. While his marriage proved no deterrent to his having extramarital sex, he thought that it did lead him to minimize the number of sexual partners. Once Henry had finished his degree and obtained his professional qualifications, he decided it was time for marriage. He too explained that he was prompted to marry largely because of what he considered his ever-increasing risk of exposure to HIV infection. He decided upon a female acquaintance, a family friend, as a likely candidate to be his wife and began inquiries into her background and suitability. Henry was satisfied with what he discovered of the young woman's character and personality and they became engaged. At his fiancée's insistence, they postponed intercourse until marriage, a condition that Henry grudgingly agreed to, though, in his account, it led to his engaging in other sexual relationships. He recalled thinking at the time, "Let me enjoy myself before I marry!" His determination to enjoy himself would not be curtailed by marriage. Most men would continue to seek sexual partners beyond their marriage. For some this meant that sexual relationships already begun with other young women continued, when chance allowed or more usually when men engineered the opportunity.

While the men claimed a Christian identity, few married in church. Mutinta was one of the minority who, in his early thirties, got married in a Catholic Church at his wife's insistence. Mutinta formerly attended a Protestant church but he was no longer a churchgoer. His study of philosophy at university had made him critical of Christian churches and those who attended them. Besides, he had read the Bible carefully and had found no black man there. He had also spent time abroad and this, together with a father who had atypically assisted in household chores and with childcare, had "opened [his] mind to many things." It had made him very critical of many aspects of life in Zambia. He particularly resented the Catholic marriage instruction he was required to attend in the weeks preceding the wedding. The majority of former students in this study had a "traditional," that is customary, village or urban wedding. They explained that the money available dictated their choice. "Traditional" weddings were cheapest. There was also the assumption that such marriages were easier to get out of, should they fail. A few men in particularly well-paid employment married in expensive civil ceremonies, costing several million kwacha. These were "European"-style "white weddings," followed by a hotel reception and, for Lusaka residents, an extended photo session either at Mundawanga Botanical Gardens south of the capital city, or beside the lake on the main university campus in Lusaka. The custom of paying *lobola* (bridewealth), which men and women called "bride-price," was universally maintained, though sometimes the full amount agreed by go-betweens in marriage negotiations had not been paid even several years after the wedding. Men who had simply started living with their wives-to-be agreed to pay a fine and those who had made their wives-to-be pregnant were often charged "damages" by the woman's family.

Former students' wives and other female family members were unanimous in their support of *lobola*. They maintained it was an important African tradition, though they recognized that the system was open to inflation and abuse. They thought it should continue in spite of commentators who cited this practice as the root of gender inequality. Payment was generally agreed to be a sign of commitment and respect for the woman and her family. As far as Sampa's mother was concerned, "Where there is no *nsalamu*, there is no marriage."[7] Some women likened the payment of *lobola* to the way white people exchanged rings. They also acknowledged that where a man was brought to a traditional court for adultery, he stood a better chance of retaining his wife if he had paid *lobola* in full. Grace, Mabvuto's wife, said she did not fully understand the point of *lobola*, "because the man takes away the woman to go and look after her." In her view, a husband should not have to pay at marriage because he will have to support his wife financially for the whole of their married life. Like other wives, however, she intended to take *lobola* for her daughters. Mabvuto had been charged four cows, though he had paid cash, at the rate of 40,000 kwacha per cow.

While many men described such payments as a sign of respect for the woman's family and as a way of "repaying" them for her upbringing and education, some also claimed that in paying *lobola* their wife had become their property. Mutinta was unique among his school contemporaries in his refusal to pay *lobola*, a custom he judged to be a meaningless superstition and a distasteful practice, "like buying someone," he explained to me. Besides, he wondered, how did families determine a just amount of money? In the event his older brother paid on his behalf. Mutinta's wife, Mutale, who was like Mutinta a university graduate, agreed with him about *lobola*. In her view, it was a tradition that had come to be abused, with parents demanding more and more money for their daughters. At best *lobola* should be no more than a small token.

Henry approached an uncle to act as intermediary in his marriage negotiations. Nominally Catholic, he arranged to marry in a Catholic Church, not, on his part, out of any religious conviction but because it was a way of inviting friends and family to join in a public celebration. However, before the wedding, in his fiancée's extended absence, Henry started a relationship with another woman Pamela. When his fiancée discovered their relationship, she called off the engagement. Henry, having made extensive inquiries about Pamela's background, in the face of criticism from his family, began marriage negotiations once more. He made a first payment toward the *lobola* that was agreed. Henry was twenty-eight when he married. He considered the custom of paying *lobola* extremely important:

> The traditional way is culturally the preferred way of doing things. If I were just to pick her and something were to happen to her, I cannot go to her people and say, "No, this is what happened," because I didn't inform them of my intentions. So if she dies, for instance, it's me to blame and I have to deal with that. I mean as far as they are concerned, their daughter is still alive. By you going through an intermediary and paying *lobola*, all that is a way of telling them, "No, this person is with me." That's a way of me having access to them to go and tell them if there is something wrong.

Pamela observed: "I have no objections to that because where I come from, when the man is charged, he first has to give something like *citenge* [a length of dress material], and when he gives cattle, the parents of the girl will say that the cattle came through the daughter."

PREGNANCY AS A PRELUDE TO MARRIAGE

The majority of the men married their wife after they became aware of her pregnancy and usually after the birth of the child. Men often gave a future wife's pregnancy as the immediate reason for deciding to marry. Though no former student explicitly stated this, it seemed as if the woman's fertility had first to be demonstrated. However, almost without exception the men described the pregnancy as an "accident," a "mistake," the consequence of "mistiming," "becoming loose," and "carelessness." A few suspected that their partners had deliberately become pregnant in order to get the men to commit themselves. Some felt trapped into marriage.

Kangwa married at the age of thirty; his wife, Catherine, was six years younger. It was not the way he had hoped and dreamed it might be in his adolescence. He had had a number of sexual partners after school and during his time at university. However, he recalled being mocked by his male age-mates because when he had completed his studies and started working he did not have a steady girlfriend. Driven by this peer pressure, he found a girlfriend. Reluctant to use condoms, he had persuaded Catherine to take contraceptive pills, insisting that the relationship was "merely for fun" and "nothing serious." Within a few months she was pregnant. Kangwa felt betrayed by Catherine. He resented the pressure put on him by her, her relatives, and his mother. After the birth of the baby, he gave in to demands from her family to enter marriage negotiations. He explained, "I felt trapped. I had told her we were just having a nice time and that it was nothing serious. I had a plan to go for further studies." He was convinced that he would never have married her, had she not got pregnant. Though the baby, in Kangwa's view, had only "the usual ailments," Catherine's parents attributed these to mystical causes associated with Kangwa's reluctance to marry and set up home together with mother and child. The baby would not be able to grow properly, they argued, without her parents living together in marriage. According to Kangwa, Catherine cynically concurred with her parents' diagnosis, though, like him, she did not in fact believe in such things. The final straw for Kangwa was when his own mother, fearing a mystical attack, also began to apply pressure:

> My mother said, "They are going to bewitch you. Or if they are not going to bewitch you, they are going to bewitch me. They will say, 'You are the one who is stopping your son from marrying our daughter.'" Anyway, I married her. We stayed together and had another child, another girl. It's now marriage!

On the completion of his university studies Paul soon found employment. He had had no fear of AIDS, but he had always dreaded making his girlfriend, Matilda, pregnant. Yet he discovered that he had been "caught off guard." Formerly Born Again, though at this period a "backslider," to his chagrin, he found that he was not beyond sin himself: he made his future wife pregnant. Paul and Matilda had thought they were being careful in their relationship, using condoms when it was not "safe" to have unprotected sex. He came to the conclusion that they had "overlooked some facts." Matilda's pregnancy depressed Paul. He felt trapped, though he concluded that he should marry her as she would be a good mother to his children. In retrospect, in his forties and now once more Born Again, he judged that the fact that he had made his girlfriend pregnant was an indication that he had "lost the right course."

At college Enoch began a relationship with a young woman that resulted in a pregnancy before the end of his first year. She already had two small children. Enoch's future mother-in-law actively encouraged the relationship. "Initially," he explained, "even when I impregnated her [made her pregnant], I had no intention of marrying her. Now, I don't know how things turn in life, if it's the mind or sympathy comes in, but I married her for the love of the child."

Atypically among his contemporaries, Malama married at the early age of twenty-one. He attributed this to the fact that he was brought up in a village where early marriage was expected; it was a product, he said, of the "village mentality." He had no regrets, quite the contrary, as he reflected on the devastation that AIDS had brought:

> In fact I think it was a blessing in disguise because when I married many of my other movements, womanizing, having sex, these things that young boys and men do, all these were monitored. And that probably explains why I am still alive now when many of my friends who didn't marry at my age—they have either died or they are just sick now, sick in bed, dying of AIDS.

However, marriage had proved no bar to extramarital sex. In Malama's estimation, during his marriage he had "not that many sexual partners, thirty at the most."

Sometimes fathers imposed their will. In his first year at college Promise made a second-year student, Susan, pregnant. She was four years younger than Promise. Susan was allowed to write her exams. After she gave birth, she happened to be posted to work close to the home of Promise's father. Promise would visit Susan and the baby when he went home to see his parents. His prolonged absences during the holidays caused his father to complain that his son had become "too movious."[8] In a chance encounter, Promise's former primary school headmaster told him, "Your son usually comes here. You have a grandson somewhere here." Promise had gone with friends on a week's hunting expedition. Back at the homestead, returning from the nearby river where he had gone to bathe, he saw his girlfriend with their baby being brought by his brother on a bicycle. His father angrily confronted him, Promise recalled: " 'Ah! Why do you fear me? Why did you not at least tell your mother?' " Promise explained that he was waiting for an appropriate moment to break the news. Promise's father asked him whether he was ready to marry Susan, but Promise said he was not. However, his father was not prepared to accept any excuses. Promise reluctantly agreed to marry if his father was prepared to pay for the marriage and to support Susan and the baby until he had finished his studies. His father came to an agreement about the payments with Susan's mother. They had a "traditional" wedding. *Litete* [sweet beer] was brewed and Promise's father slaughtered a cow. When he was posted to the south of the country, his father insisted that Susan and the child go with him, explaining to Susan, " 'Where he is going there are women. He might marry there, so go with him!' "

Hambayi married at twenty-three. His father forced him into the decision while assuring financial support. Hambayi had started working and had become attracted to a grade nine schoolgirl, Rebecca. The marriage was not planned. He explained to me that he was simply "playing with" (having sex with) her. Having spent the night with him, Rebecca had overslept and missed school. Her parents complained. They told him he should keep the girl as he had "abducted" her and therefore "married" her. Hambayi thought he had no alternative but to marry Rebecca. There was no ceremony as the matter was considered a case of elopement. Hambayi paid her parents 600 kwacha (approximately half of his yearly earnings at the time). Despite his anger, Hambayi's father contributed some of the money. Hambayi paid the rest with money he received from the sale of one of his eight head of cattle.

Recovering from his third episode of venereal disease, Sampa decided that he should marry "for safety reasons." It would prove unreliable insurance as he continued to have unprotected sex with a number of women. He was thirty-one when he married for the first time. He met his first wife, Mulenga, at his shebeen. His wife-to-be, two years younger than him, was from his ethnic group; she was living in the same compound. After they had started a sexual relationship, Sampa became concerned that other men would approach her for sex: "I told her, 'No, you can't be staying where we drink beer because a lot of men will be coming. They will be doing to you the same that I am doing to you.' So I found another house away from the shebeen." At first he had no intention of marrying her, but he came around to the idea, he explained, "She's not bad. She's beautiful!" There was no marriage ceremony. Sampa said that he "just picked her" and they started living together. He agreed to pay the 200,000 kwacha *lobola* that Mulenga's parents demanded. Sampa considered the payment very important, a sign to her parents that he had accepted their daughter as his wife. He also commented that paying *lobola* was "like you are buying that lady. She becomes your property. (Laughing.) She belongs to you. She's subjected to you."

With the exception of Mutinta, former students who in many respects considered themselves to be "modern" men still claimed the importance of the "tradition" of *lobola*. For some, this was because it seemed to confirm a sense of ownership over their wives. However, beyond this, it was clear that men considered that propriety required them to act in this way. As in the area of sexuality, most saw the payment of bridewealth as a quintessential expression of an African identity that set them apart and from which, in this context, they could derive a sense of pride.

The Importance of Children

From childhood the men interviewed had been anxious to prove their masculinity, and thereby qualify for adult male status, through the production of children. The birth of children changed many men's sense of themselves in the world. They believed others perceived them differently, especially once marriage accorded them the respect due to husbands who were also fathers. Within the household, husbands and wives often used teknonyms as forms of address, speaking to and referring to one another as "Mother of" and "Father of" their named first-born child. Men repeatedly invoked God as the giver of children who were a blessing. However, there were several instances in which men assisted their premarital and extramarital sexual partners to have abortions. Sometimes men's wives were aware of the other children men had fathered in premarital and extramarital relationships and sometimes they were not. There were instances where a man clandestinely continued a sexual relationship with the mother of one of his children while married to another woman. Indeed, some men claimed that partners from previous relationships remained sexually available to them, even if the women themselves were married to other men. Some married couples experienced the pain of a still birth or repeated miscarriages. And yet, a "real man" must produce children; any man who did not came under openly critical scrutiny. Once married, men reported particularly intense pressure from their mothers to provide them with grandchildren.

When a marriage did not produce children in the first or second year, some men blamed their wives for "failing" to give them children and sought divorce. "Traditionally, you have to have children," Sampa chuckled. "You have to leave your image. For me, it's important to leave my image. Others will look at your child and remember you, 'Oh, at one time lived so-and-so!'" Two years after marrying Mulenga, Sampa became concerned because she appeared unable to become pregnant. He tried to discover the cause. He was driven to do this, he explained, in part because he felt bad about his workmates' taunts, "Big as you are and you don't have a baby?" Both men and women were, he said, "laughing at" him, adding, "You know, such things are very difficult in our society. Someone who's married and they don't have a baby!"[9] In fact, unknown to them, and to his wife, he was fairly sure that he had recently fathered a child with one of his girlfriends at work. He persuaded his wife to have a gynecological examination. He had tests to determine his sperm count, which, he reported, was "excellent." Sampa decided he needed to find another wife to have children with. He became attracted to a young woman, Ruth, who was ten years his junior. She had left school after grade nine and was working in the restaurant where he usually had his lunch. Within a few weeks, Sampa proposed marriage, explaining that he wanted to leave his current wife as she could not give him children. Ruth said she would consider his proposal. They had not had sexual intercourse at this stage. One Friday evening, Sampa took her—she thought for drinks—to a hotel. His intention was to have sex with her. He drank some beers because, he explained to me, he was "a bit shy," and he plied her with brandy. He then took her to a room that he had booked for the night. The following day, arriving at her home in a taxi, they were confronted by Ruth's mother who refused them entry. They decided to return to the hotel where they spent the rest of the weekend. On Monday morning Mulenga arrived at Sampa's workplace and caused a scene, mistakenly accusing one of his girlfriends at work of having spent the weekend with him. She was persuaded to return home and to try and settle the problem there.

Within a short while Sampa told Mulenga that Ruth was pregnant. In Sampa's account Mulenga tried to trick him into thinking that she too was pregnant. Sampa, assisted by his female cousin, discovered traces of the telltale signs of what they decided was Mulenga's menstruation. When they confronted her, Mulenga claimed that she had miscarried. Sampa refused to believe her and decided to marry Ruth. Mulenga was prepared to stay in a polygamous marriage. However, Sampa explained that though his father was a polygamist, he thought he was too young and too poor to have two wives. It did not appeal to him and besides, expressing a commonly held fear among men, he explained to me that he was afraid that his first wife might poison him. Moreover, Ruth's family would not allow her to move into the household while Mulenga was still in residence. In negotiations with Ruth's uncle, Sampa agreed to pay her family 250,000 kwacha *lobola*. He made a first payment of 50,000 kwacha. There was no ceremony, Sampa explained, because he had already made Ruth pregnant.

At nineteen, Edward, almost uniquely among his school contemporaries, did not think that having children was so important. However, at forty he had grown aware of the envy of others. He described the pressure he felt he had come under to become a father. His first marriage ended in divorce because his wife did not become pregnant:

> I lived with my wife for three years but everybody was asking why I was not having a child. They would ask, "How come?" My parents started bothering me, especially my mum, my uncles and elder sisters. I told them that I didn't marry in order to have children. Even friends would be asking during beer drinking whether or not I had a child. You see, in the compound, I was the only one who went to school [university]—and I was married to a rich man's daughter. So people wanted to spot my weaknesses. In the fifth year of our marriage, the pressure on my wife was too much. We began to consult doctors but I found it to be a nuisance. We consulted a herbalist from Zimbabwe. We were losing money for nothing. My wife started to bring home all sorts of medicines. I would confiscate the herbs, but she complained and asked me to take her back to her parents. We decided to divorce.... Pressure continued from my family. When I was found doing laundry, I would be told to marry. I would be called *nkungulume* [bachelor]. My family would not come to my home because they said there was nobody to cook for them.... Later I married again. I got to know my wife when she was a schoolgirl. Now that I am a father I have proved a lot of people wrong.

Simon was still unmarried in 2002 (as he would be in 2008). At nineteen, he had given no thought to marriage—which he imagined would be many years hence—or to what qualities a future wife might possess. After university, Simon had a number of girlfriends. One relationship had lasted for seven years and Simon had hoped that it might lead to marriage. However, his partner had gone abroad to study and when he went to visit her, he discovered that she had joined a religious cult that only permitted sex between cult members. Another relationship resulted in a child, though the baby died soon after birth. Simon tried to use condoms in all his relationships. He was opposed to the idea of having an unplanned pregnancy. At times, however, he had unprotected sex. He described his behavior on such occasions as "stupid." He interpreted his actions as the result of depression and anger. At times he had had no condoms with him and had been "silly and gone down the line of erotic stimulation and then got to the point of no turning back." At almost forty years of age, Simon, the (publicly) childless bachelor, was under constant pressure from family members, friends, and work colleagues, who were suspicious about this failure to achieve male adulthood. They wanted him to marry and "settle down." Though they respected his success and appreciated the material assistance he could give them, his bachelor status troubled them. Several of his female relatives asked me to encourage him to marry. His mother spoke unhappily to me about his sexual relationships with women, commenting, "He should stop spoiling other people's daughters." Simon assumed that all the questions about when he might marry from his uncles and aunts were prompted by his mother. He managed to laugh them off and give them, he said, "all sorts of excuses." Some of them had met one or two of his girlfriends and this had apparently put their fears to rest. Simon explained: "Maybe they thought that I couldn't have an erection. Well, I don't know whether they thought it to that extent. But it was something I thought about, so I said, 'Well, it's not that.'"

Marriage Instruction

Most wives had received some instruction when they first menstruated (*cisungu*) from midwives and women elders (in Bemba, *banacimbusa*) about the care of the body and the dangers of sex before marriage. All the wives of former students received further instruction from *banacimbusa* immediately prior to marriage, though the duration and extent of teaching varied considerably.[10] In contrast, men's instructions prior to marriage were perfunctory. Several men and women recalled that elders had taught them that between husband and wife there were many secrets that should never be revealed to others. Brides-to-be were given this admonition with particular force.[11] Like many of his school contemporaries, Promise recalled how, at his customary marriage, elders gave the couple advice separately and together. In instructions apart from his wife, Promise remembered his grandfather and other male elders advising him never to beat his wife: "They also said that the only way that you could be loved and stay with your wife was to have sex with her. If you don't have sex with your wife, she will think you are going out with other ladies." If his wife accused him of extramarital affairs, he was to deny everything:

> When I got married, well I was told, in our African tradition, if you happen to go out with [have sex with] a lady, outside marriage that is, say your wife comes and finds you on top of that lady. On top of that lady! Don't accept! [Don't admit it!] No, don't accept! You, you continue saying "No." If you say "Yes," that means that you have lost interest in your wife. And that wife of yours will say, "No, this person doesn't love me." So the best way, even if your wife sees you, just say, "No! I haven't done it."

Young women were instructed to follow the traditions of the past as maintained "in the village," that is the rural areas, as opposed to what was found in town, where many adopted "modern" white ways. The white "European" world was often a target for censure, as one mother, and *banacimbusa*, commented:

> Today's young people—in the towns especially—have no respect for tradition. Young girls are wearing mini-skirts and trousers. However, young people from the village have respect. In our time we were told that if a man proposes love it should mean marriage and not sex. We abstained in our time. These days young people want to behave like *bazungu* [white people]. Too many videos are contributing to this.... These days the girls will have had sex even before they are brought for lessons [marriage instruction]. They have learnt a lot in the discos and on channel "O" on television.

At the heart of the lessons was the need for a wife to give her husband respect. Several wives recalled that they had been instructed that once their husband called them, they had to answer "*Baba*" [Father]. Wives-to-be learnt what their duties should entail. A wife should rise early to prepare a bath for the husband and make his breakfast. She should be brave and persevere. She should ignore rumors about her husband's extramarital affairs. She should "fear" (respect) her husband and never ask him why he came home late. She should learn how to read her husband's moods. She should avoid quarrels and never act on impulse. She should never show anger toward her husband. If her husband made a mistake, he would eventually admit it. In a marriage one person had to be humble and that should be the woman. Some women were taught that when a man beat his wife, especially a slap or two, this was a sign of his love for her. A woman must not complain at the first beating. However, if it got out of hand, she should run to her husband's relatives because these were the people who knew him best and would be able to handle him. If the woman ran to her parents, there would be war between the families. If this did not solve the problem, she should seek help from her church. Men who did not go to church were a particular problem. Some wives deserved to be beaten, especially those who neglected household chores. However, some wives-to-be were also warned that men only beat their wives when other women with whom they were having affairs were using *muti* (medicine) on them. Brides-to-be were told to abstain from sex when they were menstruating, because the forefathers said it was not good to have intercourse during this time.[12] A wife should never let her husband see her menstrual blood. The pieces of cloth used by women during her menstruation must be kept away from the man. It was possible that some men might use them to make their own charms.

While children were essential to the maintenance of a marriage, young women were instructed about contraceptives, both pills and injections, because it was important that childbirth should be spaced. Most brides-to-be were well acquainted with contraceptive options. Some midwives warned that extended use of the pill might lead to long-term infertility. Some women were told to allow husbands to ejaculate between the thighs when they were pregnant. Condoms did not figure in marriage instruction as they were judged to encourage "promiscuity." Condoms were "for the bar" not for the home. Besides, some women were told by *banacimbusa* that they provided no protection from HIV.

When a husband came home from drinking, he should find food ready for him. A wife must be a good cook, varying the relish she prepared and choosing for her husband the parts of meat that he most enjoyed. He should be given whatever he demanded—especially sex. He should never be refused. Men needed frequent sexual intercourse and could not go for more than a few days without sex. Women were taught how to satisfy their husbands sexually. Some young women were said to be "too difficult" and this was given as an explanation why their husbands sought other women. Indeed, instructors taught the brides-to-be that "marriage is sex." If the woman did not "give in" to her husband's demands, the man would "starve" and start going for other women. A young wife should never ask for sex or tell her husband if she was not satisfied sexually. She should be too shy to do so. While wives recognized their role as one of care for their husbands, few were prepared to follow this last injunction. Several women received both "traditional" and "Christian" teaching—at times from the same instructress. Mukuka's wife recalled the instruction she received at her Pentecostal church before marriage:

> There were things I did not know. For example, I did not know that we have to have sex nearly every day. I was told that I have to show respect for my mother-in-law because she is also my mother. I was told to be submissive to my husband since the Bible says so as well. I was told the man is the head of the house. I have to love him, to obey him and to be humble. I have to have respect for him no matter what happens. I was taught how to look after a man. I have to wash his clothes so that he looks nice. As for his duties, my husband has to love me, to provide for the family and for me, his wife. He should satisfy me in bed as well.

The secret of marriage was not herbs but cleanliness. Young women were taught how to keep their bodies and their homes clean. A wife must wash and iron her husband's clothes properly. She should welcome her husband's relatives, showing them respect, giving them food, smiling and laughing with them. She must ignore any insults from her husband's family. While the woman should do all she could to please her husband, she was taught that he, in his turn, should make sure that his wife was satisfied; he should provide whatever his wife needed. Men were "naturally difficult." They might be taught how to behave, but they often failed to follow what they had learnt. Young men were a particular problem because they thought that what they learnt from elders was old-fashioned. However, there were some men who loved their wives so much that they would even do household chores when their wives were sick.

Many mothers and grandmothers who helped prepare young women for marriage were critical of young women.[13] Some thought their abandonment of tradition was the cause of HIV/AIDS. Despite ethnographies that demonstrate that in the early- and mid-twentieth century virginity was neither valued nor expected among Bemba- and Tonga-speaking people (Richards 1982: 158; Colson 1958: 289), older women insisted that in their youth premarital sex *of any kind* was forbidden. While older women insisted that this was African tradition, such claims might well be a consequence of mission Christianity that condemned any form of premarital sexual activity as sinful and uncivilized. (See Jeater 1993.)

Some brides were brought to their husbands wearing beads around their waist that husbands could fondle. Many men found beads on a naked woman sexually arousing. Some beads were known to have been treated with *muti* (medicine) to make the woman's body warm and inviting. However, several *banacimbusa*, especially those who belonged to Pentecostal churches, emphasized that they did not give *muti* to their pupils. The only medicine in marriage was respect, respect for one's husband and respect for oneself. The caring role that was expected of wives and the implied exchange relationship in marriage were at times acted out during wedding ceremonies, as described by a Lusaka-based instructress originally from Eastern Province:

> The girl will come dancing to the man's home. This is followed by shaving. Then the woman puts the man on her lap and feeds him with *nsima* (maize porridge). The two are stark naked in the bedroom. The man must be fed with two lumps only—the same way we feed a child. After that the outside and the inside of the man's mouth is cleaned by the woman. This is followed by making the man drink some of the sweet beer that has been brought. The man still remains in the lap of the woman. Again he only drinks twice and then he is cleaned. The woman will then clap her hands. The full *nsima* will be eaten after the man has been bathed by his wife-to-be. He is bathed slowly and he pays some money.

Cleaning after Sex

In many respects, wives became their husbands' teachers, instructing them how to follow "African tradition" in sexual matters. Wives, whatever their ethnic group, had been taught by their women instructors that it was their duty to clean their husband's penis after sexual intercourse.[14] Wives should have at least two handkerchiefs or other pieces of cloth for cleaning, which should be kept hidden. The performance of this task was the clearest expression of respect and care for a husband. Cleaning a husband's penis signaled legitimate sexual intercourse. The burden of maintaining the purity of the marriage lay firmly with the wives. However, former students and their wives dismissed any fears of mystical harm from the nonobservance of such practices.[15] Many men had initially been surprised to discover that their wife was expected to clean them after sex. Although several said they did not like it or felt embarrassed at first, when told it was "tradition," they accepted this practice.

Men offered me several interpretations of the practice of cleaning. Many suggested it was purely for hygiene. While a few men said that they were not against cleaning their wives, they explained that anatomical differences made it an unnecessary or difficult task. Most former students, however, did not consider that a husband should clean his wife.[16] They maintained it was a demonstration of men's "superiority," explaining that the wife's act of cleaning was a sign of her submission, of her inferior status. Dominic was one of those who interpreted his wife cleaning him in this way:

> As for myself, I do respect tradition. It's important. I am an African and these things have been passed on from generation to generation.... These things were put there by people who thought that this is the best we can do. My wife cleans me. For me to clean her would have no meaning, but for her to clean me, it's part of making my wife very subordinate. The way I look at it, after having sex, you make the woman clean that white stuff—it's part of making the woman very submissive.

Like other men, Mabvuto spoke of a wife cleaning her husband as "a traditional rule" that must be followed. While he denied that he ever cleaned his wife, Grace, she said that he occasionally did so. Some men expected all the women they had sex with to clean them. Promise had been taught in marriage instructions that his wife should clean his penis after sex, and then clean herself. He did not know the reason for this practice, but readily accepted this "tradition" and had never wondered about its purpose. He expected other women he had sex with to do the same: "Sometimes I have to tell them, but most of these ladies who have undergone initiation, you don't have to tell them. They just do it. You don't need to tell the woman. She knows by herself, 'I have to do this.' "

Darius, like Promise, expected all the women he had sex with to clean him. "It is something I have culturally inherited," he explained. "Those ladies sit down with their parents when they are growing up and they are taught what to do for us men." However, several men told me that they did not allow extramarital partners to clean them because they were afraid that they risked being bewitched. The ambivalent power of sex was clear. (See Heald 1995.) Women, normally said to be subservient, could then also act in a threatening manner. Here, as elsewhere, despite appearances, power was not all in one direction. Sampa, for example, felt that other women should not handle his penis as they would learn too much about him; besides, they might use his semen to lure him away from his wife. In rare instances a man refused to allow his wife to clean him, explaining that he found it embarrassing and unnecessary. Some men stated that, while there were times when they might clean themselves after sex, it remained a wife's duty to clean them. Others appeared indifferent, claiming that the practice was maintained at their wife's insistence. Malama explained, "My wife cleans me after sex. To me it doesn't matter, but it matters to her. It's like that is what she was taught during her initiation." Peter, an exception in this as in so many matters, cleaned his wife after sexual intercourse. He explained that his wife, for religious reasons, had not received any instruction on this matter and so, in Peter's words, "We teach one another." He saw their mutual cleaning as an expression of care and love.

Shaving

While cleaning was generally not reciprocal, regular reciprocal shaving of body hair, particularly pubic hair, was a feature of married life. Wives shaved their husbands and were shaved by them in turn. Hygiene was advanced by men and women as the reason for this activity; hair was said to be dirty and, especially on a man's body, a sign of neglect. Shaving, an expression of care, also had erotic potential and often led to intercourse. Women placed particular importance on shaving, aware of cases brought against wives whose husbands had been discovered to be unshaven. "Death is common these days," they observed. A husband should always be shaved regularly. If he died and his relatives discovered long pubic hair, they would accuse his widow of neglect or worse. Stella, Paul's sister, noted the asymmetry in these requirements: "If my husband died today with pubic hair, my family will be fined. His family will say that I didn't care for him, but if I die with my pubic hair, well, there is nothing that will be said about it."

Each partner might shave themselves, with the permission of the other, but shaving without permission constituted "a case," arousing suspicions of infidelity. Malama explained, "We do shave one another—the body, the private parts. If I shaved myself, that would cause uproar.... That would bring a lot of confusion because she would take it that I was shaved by some other person."

Mabvuto insisted on the importance of husband and wife shaving one another: "When it comes to shaving, the husband has to shave the wife as well. If I find that my wife's parts have been shaved, it is an offence because she has to inform me or ask me to shave her. Shaving herself without my consent is not advisable." Sampa accepted mutual shaving as an important tradition. It was what he was taught when he married, though he could find no reason for it. In his marriage it was almost always a prelude to intercourse. He and his wife normally shaved one another every couple of weeks. He understood the practice to be "just a matter of cleanliness—nothing else," commenting, "This is my culture." If she were to discover on her return from a prolonged absence that his pubic hair was shaven, her suspicions of his infidelity would be confirmed and it would constitute "a big case." When his wife was busy, with her permission, he might shave himself under his armpits when he bathed, but, he explained, "as for the private parts—she has to do it!" One of his girlfriends had wanted to shave him; despite her tears, he had rejected her offer. He was conscious that this would immediately signal to his wife that he had been unfaithful to her. He would draw similar conclusions himself, if he discovered that his wife had been shaved without his doing so.

Darius was one of the few men to reject the idea that a husband was responsible for shaving his wife. He appeared ambivalent about the practice, a custom that seemed to suggest to him a lack of "civilization," though he also related it to the need for women to show their care for men: "It is awkward, but despite having gone through school and civilization we have inherited this. A woman looks at the man like her own property. She has to take care of the man otherwise somebody else will take care of the man."

Henry had long refused to allow his wife, Pamela, to shave him. However, a case arose when one of Henry's uncles died and was discovered to have long pubic hair. Pamela seized the opportunity to complain to one of Henry's aunts about his reluctance. Faced with their combined protestations, he agreed to submit to being regularly shaved. Peter understood the requirement of a wife to shave her husband's pubic and other body hair to be a "traditional" practice. In his home they only did this when he wanted it. In general, he and his wife shaved themselves. Peter explained that his Seventh Day Adventism had caused him to depart from "tradition." He had not found such practices in the Bible.

Conclusion

Almost all men reported greater sexual activity after school with increasing numbers of sexual partners. They spoke of the period as a time when they became "loose." Many of them sought out schoolgirls for casual sex, or for long-term relationships in exchange for financial support. Several men met their wives in this way. With some exceptions, they continued to exercise their preference for unprotected sex even when they had much easier access to condoms than they had had during their schooldays and even though information about HIV/AIDS was becoming increasingly available. In time, however, HIV/AIDS became a catalyst for many in their decision to marry; having a wife at home would, they reasoned, render the need for other sexual partners unnecessary. In few households did this subsequently prove to be the case.

Throughout the extended period of premarital sexual activity, young men felt threatened by women whom they feared might give them HIV. Yet none of them considered that they might be just as likely to transmit HIV to their sexual partners. With a few exceptions, what exercised their minds was the peer pressure they might face, should they fail to gain the accoutrements of successful male adulthood: first a girlfriend, or girlfriends, and later a wife and children.

In observing the customs of *lobola*, of shaving their wives and being cleaned after sex, men claimed the importance of "tradition." Sex, for many of them, became a primary arena in which they came to know themselves as "African." (See chapter 6.) Potent semen, once ejaculated, rapidly became "dirt" that a subservient wife should clean away. In this instance the power of the Bemba wife symbolized in the marriage pot and described by Richards (1982) had been usurped by her husband. Formerly, she alone could purify her husband after sex and protect him, their children, and others from mystical harm. While former students and their wives denied such harm was possible, the "traditional" practice in a different form was maintained by almost all of them. But now many men interpreted the requirement of wives to clean them as a sign of women's inferiority. Nevertheless, in intimate matters, wives became their husbands' instructors in the proper conduct of marital sex. In the privacy of sexual relationships, a man's claim to be the dominant partner was undermined. While ready to take up the role of carers, providing husbands with the comforts of home, young women were not totally submissive, *pace* the stress placed in marriage instruction upon the need for a wife's humility. Especially with regard to sexual satisfaction, contrary to what many had been taught, they were determined that their own desires should be made known and fulfilled. The complex ambiguities of male-female relationships in marriage found expression in "traditional" teachings when a woman was instructed to call her husband "*Baba*," while, paradoxically being told that a man was merely a child and a man's wife had to be his mother.[17]

5

Married Life

Unaware of their HIV status before marriage, many of the men in this study envisaged that married life would prove a powerful prophylactic against AIDS; when they wanted to have sex, they would turn to their wives instead of "hunting for women." However, most continued to have unprotected sex with multiple partners. There was almost no communication between husband and wife regarding a husband's extramarital affairs and the risk of HIV infection. Among their wives, as among Zambian women more generally, a commonly expressed sentiment was "A marriage certificate is often a death certificate." Wives assumed that husbands engaged in unprotected sex and that even if the men used condoms, they doubted they could prevent AIDS. While most felt unable to confront their husbands with their well-founded anxieties, this did not render them powerless in *all* aspects of their lives. Men and women were variously situated in shifting fields of power. No simplistic portrayal of an all-encompassing patriarchy will suffice to give an adequate account of quotidian married life.

The comprehensive ethnographies by Audrey Richards and Elizabeth Colson provide rich insights into rural Bemba and Tonga gender relations and marriage in the colonial period. In her analysis, Colson noted that the Tonga man had exclusive possession of his wife but this was not reciprocated. She reported that the majority of her informants considered religious labels to be of little importance and suggested that while missionary condemnation of premarital affairs seemed to carry little weight, increased prosperity appeared to lead to an increase in "promiscuity" among young men (1958: 291–293). Richards suggested that companionship in Bemba marriages, where it existed, was something of a "happy accident" (Richards 1969: 23). Moore and Vaughan (1994: 171), in their critical reassessment of Richard's work, have argued that by the 1950s a shift in the balance of power between partners had occurred. Changes brought about largely through men's labor migration to urban centers meant that it was now women, rather than men, who needed to be married.

Anthropologists of urban marriage in the colonial and postcolonial periods have offered a very bleak picture. Powdermaker characterized 1950s marriage on the Copperbelt as relationships of "distrust and jealousy" (1962: 151) and Epstein, writing of the same region and period, spoke of the "canker of distrust" (1981: 121) between men and women. Schuster's sensationalist account declared Lusaka marriages to be in a "pathological" condition (1979: 130). In her longitudinal study of low-income households in Mtendere, a Lusaka compound, Hansen highlighted the manner in which "women and men [were] grappling about how conjugal life should be structured in a situation of tension" (1996: 120). She noted wives' suspicions and the fact that they did not expect to have their husbands' undivided attention either economically or sexually, and the degree to which sexuality continued to be a key dimension of women's identity. Ferguson reported that, in his fieldwork on the Zambian Copperbelt in the mid- and late 1980s, he found domestic life among miners "remarkably similar" to that described by Powdermaker and Epstein, a context in which relations were "shifting and sexually plural" (1999: 187). However, Ferguson argued that a political economy of misogyny and antagonism became intelligible because of the overwhelming predicament of economic decline in which women suffered most from fierce male resentment. If anything, "hostility and mutual suspicion" seemed to Ferguson to have intensified: "It was expected that both married men and women would have many sexual partners.... While the threat of AIDS was much on men's minds...few regarded it as a legitimate reason to forego these affairs (or to use condoms which were in any case not widely available)" (ibid.). Men, Ferguson observed, considered sexual exclusion "unnatural" and declared himself unprepared for "the intensity of working men's misogyny." Rude (1999) explored Zambian men's violence toward women by examining the outcomes of court cases from the 1970s to the 1990s that were reported in Zambian newspapers. She argued that media coverage and judicial comments reflected myths and misinformation about domestic violence and homicide where women were portrayed as provoking "reasonable" men to use violence against them. In this way male violence was seen as predictable and largely acceptable.

The Question of Trust in Former Students' Marriages

Unlike the trust between sons and mothers that former students reported in adolescence, and, with few exceptions, in adulthood, marital relationships were generally marked by distrust. Several men said they trusted no one. While wives often expressed distrust of their husbands, very few spoke to them directly about this. Ironically, the majority of the men in this study described women as "naturally trusting." Simon, like others, acknowledged that double standards applied:

> I think the men trust the women but at the slightest hint of something—that the woman has gone out [had extramarital sex] or something—then, he gives her a big beating. I think to a great extent that the women know that the men are not to be trusted, but it is something that they learn to live with. But the men, if they learn about it, well, they really get mad about it. I mean if men find out that their wives are messing around, well, they divorce them immediately. To them it seems like this is a sign of weakness on them, a sign of their weakness to their family. It looks like a sign to the man's family that he can't control the woman, his wife.... They will go and get a new woman who they think is faithful, even though they are not necessarily being faithful themselves.

Extramarital affairs were one means by which some former students showed their peers that they were not under their wives' control. Some men also explained to me that they feared that other women would question their manhood if they did not try to have sex with them. They described their extramarital activity as "misbehaving." Several men suggested to me that extramarital sex was a marked feature of "African sexuality." To demonstrate to other men, and at times to other family members, that they were not "under petticoat government," on leaving home, many men would not say where they were going or when they might return. (See Hansen 1996: 127 for similar observations.) In contrast, women constantly reported their movements beyond the household, to their husbands if they were at home, and sometimes to me, in their husbands' absence. Few couples displayed what they described as "English manners," where husband and wife could be seen to enjoy a companionable relationship beyond the confines of the home.

Joshua offered his own explanation for the absence of trust between husbands and wives. He felt frustrated by the corruption in public life. "The danger with Zambians is not only at the level of the home," he commented. "We can't trust even our President. Because you are suspicious of what other people are doing you can also be suspicious of what your wife is doing." Joshua had been retrenched. He found other work as a laborer but his monthly income was more than halved, from as much as 1 million kwacha (about U.S. $220), with overtime, to 300,000 kwacha (about U.S. $70). Joshua and his wife, Sarah, struggled to make ends meet. Sarah was in poor health and had no paid employment. After paying for electricity and water, the couple were left with very little for food and other expenses for themselves, their five children, and a nephew and niece, both orphaned by AIDS, whom they looked after. The couple had managed to buy their own house, though it was now in a poor state of repair. Joshua's pay went straight into the bank and he gave his wife his payslip. Sarah made all withdrawals from their joint account and controlled all household spending. Joshua felt enormous pressure to live up to the essential requirement of the "real man," that is, to provide for his family. He often spoke of his sense of inadequacy. He had married Sarah after he made her pregnant. He was twenty-three years old and was working as an apprentice. Sarah was seventeen and in grade ten at secondary school. Her pregnancy ended her formal education. Men like Joshua, who stayed home most of the time when not at work, and who informed their wives about their movements, were subject to ridicule by both men and women. Joshua observed:

> People go round saying that when a man stays at home it means that a woman must have applied some herbs to keep the man at home. The woman must have done something. It is something my wife has several times come to say to me. People tell her, "Your husband is always at the church. If he is not at church he is at home or with that one friend of his. What have you given him? What have you done to him?"[1]

In contrast to Joshua, Paul was among the most successful of his school contemporaries. His take-home pay was around 7 million kwacha (U.S. $1550). In addition, he enjoyed various company perks. He had taken on a substantial mortgage to buy his house. Despite his salary, Paul felt under constant pressure from his siblings (three of whom lived with him) and extended family members who looked to him for support. As in other marriages, tensions arose when his wife Matilda considered that he was assisting his relatives to the detriment of their three children's well-being. Matilda had no paid employment. She suspected Paul was having an extramarital affair and asked me to speak "indirectly" to him about the risk of HIV infection. However, Paul was one of the minority of his contemporaries who said he had complete trust in his wife. He offered an idealized portrait of past village life and argued that trust *between men* had been considered essential. In a Bemba village the proven liar (in Bemba *uwabufi*) faced exclusion from village affairs. Paul suggested that modernity had brought with it an absence of trust among men and between men and women. Born Again, he pondered long and hard when I asked him to name the people he felt he could trust—as the following interview extract illustrates:

TONY: Who do you trust?

(Long pause.) (Silence.)

PAUL: It's a very difficult question.... The word of God says, "Do not put your trust in man"... Who do I trust? Well, I think I trust God. But apart from that I do trust other people. I (laughing) I trust my mother. I mean—what do I mean? (Pause.) I don't mean that she can do everything that I ask. I mean she will do that which she intends to do. She'll do her best to do it. I trust my wife. I think she is quite sincere even when she's ignorant or she's angry or she's wrong, I trust her. You know, with her human failings. I trust her. I cherish her. She's a person I can rely upon.... And, well, this can be considered very subjective because you are interviewing me, but I think I can trust you. I am able to say things to you that I wouldn't say to many other people. I can trust you because I, well, humanly speaking, you've been fairly consistent in our relationship. I mean, so, to put it crudely, you have earned my trust. So to speak, you've earned your trust with me, although we don't say it like that, in a sense as we grow in a relationship we do earn each other's trust, whether willingly or unwillingly. I mean, it just comes as a consequence of past events. So I don't know many people who I trust. I trust my best friend. He's basically a trustworthy person.... I can't say I trust my boss at work. I can't say I trust most of my subordinates. I have to keep checking on them because, most of them, they don't seem to be sincere.

Ruth, Sampa's wife, like Matilda found it extremely difficult to trust her husband. In conversations with me, Sampa judged that married life had curtailed his extramarital activity. He had had no more than ten extramarital partners since his second marriage. He said he loved the other women, but insisted that they were simply "helping" him with his "sexual desire." He loved his wife and, despite disagreements, he hoped to maintain his marriage, but when he and his wife were separated he found it impossible to stay without sex week after week. He had met most of his extramarital partners in the course of his work and had given them gifts in the form of his company's products and, at times, money. While with most of the women he had had unprotected sex, he considered that he had usually safeguarded himself from the risk of disease by having sex with only a certain "class" of women—not those he called "bitches," that is, "prostitutes." In unprotected sex with those women who were not "respectable" and "decent," Sampa attributed his behavior to the influence of beer and blamed the women for not insisting on condoms. In several of the few encounters when he had used condoms, though condoms had burst, he had continued to ejaculation.

Ruth and Sampa's relationship deteriorated when he began to take part in local politics. Apart from his bringing very little money into the household, his extended absences from home caused his wife to suspect—quite rightly, though she had no firm evidence—that he was having sex with other women. In interviews, Ruth spoke of her anxieties:

> I don't know what happens at the bars. Sometimes he [Sampa] comes back home at awkward times. Well, *he* trusts me because even when he goes away, I always remain at home because I have nowhere to go. The only time I go away from home is when I go to church functions. These days are frightening because there is AIDS. It is frightening to us married women especially. You see women going about their lives, looking healthy when in actual fact they are ill. You discover that their husbands have died of AIDS.

She said she had not felt able to speak directly to her husband about her fears; however, for short periods when his absences from home caused her to suspect he had other sexual partners, she persuaded him to use condoms.[2] Sampa attributed Ruth's reluctance to seek a divorce to "tradition":

> Wives know that husbands have other women but they stay. They have respect for their husbands. I mean my wife is not supposed to ask what I am doing. A wife is not equal to the husband. I mean a man is always above a woman, always! It is not in order for a wife to bother a man about other girlfriends. You know in the north we say, "*Ubucende bwamwaume tabonaula nganda,*" "Sex outside marriage for a man does not break the relationship."[3] It's a proverb. But as for us men, immediately you hear that your wife has actually been screwed by another man, you chase her. But women, they don't even bother if they know their husband is outside the home drinking with other women. Ah, they don't say anything. It's not that they accept but they respect, "No, I shouldn't bother my husband about what he is doing with other women." But as for the woman, ah, she can never do that!

However, Sampa acknowledged that within his marriage he did not have everything his own way. In his account, Ruth was the one who decided the frequency of intercourse, though he insisted on an alternative when this was denied him:

> Well, you know, this thing of demanding sex in your house every day. So she tells you, "Ah, no, this is not the way you do these things." You see these ladies, like my wife, they are principled about having sex in the house. I mean, maybe she tells you three times a week. I mean we discuss. But mind you, in your case, you want sex every day. So like, okay, my wife I trusted her very much. Okay, if she refuses then she uses another method. I mean if she refuses me [does not allow me] to screw her, she uses another method—I mean by sucking me and I ejaculate just like that. I'm satisfied. So she was telling me, "What if I don't do these things? So you mean that you can go to some other women?" So maybe you start laughing, "Ah, that's why I've told you to do these things to me!"

Ruth had stopped work, at Sampa's insistence, soon after they set up home in the compound. She was clear about the roles of husband and wife. The husband should decide the number and the spacing of their children. Ruth expected Sampa to provide for the family, she explained: "The job of the man is to look after the welfare of the family and the education of the children. The woman's job is to ensure food is prepared, to prepare children when going to school, and to make sure the husband's clothes are clean and that the husband is properly dressed." Sampa brought his wage home and the couple sat together to decide on the household budget. Ruth commented that Sampa, as husband, had "the most power to decide." With the money available to her, Ruth made most of the decisions about food. She thought that it was Sampa's duty to discipline the children. They had two children and Sampa had decided that they could not afford to have any more. While they had access to mains electricity, water was bought at 100 kwacha per 20-liter container and the family shared a pit latrine with several neighbors. Sampa was well known in the neighborhood. While he enjoyed day-to-day life in the compound, he and his wife worried about the effect of the high level of violence and drunkenness on their young children. The family home was near several bars and shebeens, drinking places where women, some as young as fifteen, offered men sex for 10,000 kwacha (about U.S. $2) with a condom and 20,000 kwacha without a condom.

Life got more difficult for Sampa and Ruth when he lost his job for a second time. Caught stealing goods, Sampa explained to me, "These days you have to earn your own salary." He started his own business but struggled to make 200,000 kwacha each month. Sampa,

Ruth, and the children moved into his mother-in-law's household. The family decided that he could save the 150,000 kwacha he was paying in rent and contribute most of it instead to the running of the larger household. They were sixteen in all in the six-room house— Sampa and his family, his brother-in-marriage (Sampa's sister-in-law's husband) and his wife and their children, his brother-in-marriage's orphaned nephew, his father-in-law and his mother-in-law, and then other family members, three girls and a boy, two of them teenagers. Sampa and Ruth had their own bedroom. Their youngest child slept in Sampa's parents-in-law's room. Their older son slept on the kitchen floor with the other young boys. Sampa rapidly concluded he was bearing a disproportionate share of household expenses, the biggest item of which was food. He was embarrassed by Ruth's complaints about their standard of living, overheard by his mother-in-law and other members of the household. Ruth left and went to live with two of her brothers who shared a house in a neighboring compound. When Sampa's attempts to persuade her to return failed, he took their children to stay with one of his stepbrothers. He returned alone to his in-laws' household, though he found his situation "very awkward." The funeral of his brother-in-marriage (Ruth's brother-in-law who had died of AIDS) required Ruth to return to the household. Sampa and Ruth tried to resolve their differences. He agreed to Ruth's suggestion that they should find somewhere else to live. He began arrangements for them to move into the partially built house left to his cousins by Sampa's maternal uncle who had also recently died of AIDS. Sampa moved first to the house, promising he would raise the 250,000 kwacha needed to buy a door and a windowpane. He explained to Ruth that he did not think it proper for them to be sleeping together in a room without a door in the shell of a house that his female cousin, her brothers, and her two young children shared with a number of paying lodgers. Sampa visited Ruth and their children, usually carrying food for them. One day Sampa discovered that his wife had left town for Lusaka apparently intent on collecting a long-standing debt from one of her aunts, her mother's sister.

Sampa was suspicious of Ruth's motives behind her trip and was aware that her family and friends were monitoring his movements. Several weeks passed without news of her. Sampa was used to having sexual intercourse at least three or four times a week and in his wife's absence he spent more and more time with two of his girlfriends. Both of them were unmarried, about ten years younger than him, and both had young children. Sampa had already established a sexual relationship with each of them prior to his wife's departure. He had discovered that his involvement in politics and his access to party T-shirts had made him attractive to women. He had asked one of the women, Lizzie, to begin a sexual relationship within a short time of meeting her at political meetings. Despite his protestations of love she initially refused him, arguing that he was married and his wife and others would blame her if they discovered their relationship. Sampa continued his advances over a period of weeks, driven, he explained to me, by her beauty and by his desire. One evening, in a drunken condition, Sampa, in his own words, "desperate for sex," went to her home and argued that the only way their friendship would be strengthened was through sex. Lizzie told him he could not have intercourse with her because she was menstruating. He offered to use condoms but she again refused. In the end she agreed to perform oral sex on him. They started having intercourse several times a week. Though at first they used condoms, they soon stopped at Sampa's request. It was not long before Sampa began to doubt that he had exclusive sexual access to Lizzie. Though she earned an income through her work as a cleaner, he wondered who was paying her rent. He decided to terminate the relationship, concluding in a phrase commonly heard among men in Zambia, "Beautiful ones we share!" Besides, some of her women neighbors knew his wife and he feared that news of the affair would get back to her. Another of his current girlfriends, Josephine, had two young children. Afraid that she might use *muti* to cause him to divorce his wife and marry her, Sampa did not let her clean him after sex. He was careful not to bathe at her house. They quarreled frequently but always made up later. Josephine accused him of simply using her for sex. Among Sampa's reasons for liking her was the fact that she was undemanding—different, he said, from other girlfriends who were always "troubling" him for money for cosmetics and clothes. He had never asked Josephine precisely what she did to earn a living, explaining to me:

> She does something in town. I don't know what it is. In fact (laughing), I don't even care. What I am interested in is that she keeps me satisfied while my wife is away. I mean in the last week or two I've been sleeping there almost every night. Just in the night. Not during the day—because during the day people might see me and go and report. Nobody should see me when I go there. Usually I don't eat when I go there. I'm going there for sex—nothing else! (Laughing.)

Three weeks after his wife's departure, Josephine told Sampa that she was pregnant. She asked him for money for an abortion.[4] While he was pondering how to respond, one evening Sampa discovered a

Peugeot car parked outside her house. Josephine later explained to him that her children's father was visiting. He wondered whether this man was in fact their father, or someone with whom she was having an affair. Either way, he decided he would use this as an "excuse" and deny responsibility for the pregnancy, even though they had not been using condoms and he was convinced that he was responsible. He suspected that Josephine had deliberately omitted to take the contraceptive pills she had agreed to take. His female cousin encouraged him not to get involved in her decision to have an abortion. Should something go amiss, no blame would be attached to him. He acted as his cousin suggested, though he hoped Josephine would have the abortion. His wife would use the fact of a child as evidence of his infidelity. Sampa commented to me, "That would bring a lot of sparks in my marriage!" (Laughing.) Josephine had the abortion without his financial or other assistance. She was quite ill afterward; yet, within a few weeks, they resumed their sexual relationship.

Sampa increasingly missed his family. In poor health, he diagnosed that the root of his illness was that he was "thinking too much" about his wife. He missed coming home late at night and finding her asleep in bed. He missed being cared for, his meals ready when he wanted them, his clothes washed, ironed, and ready to wear. In his deceased uncle's house he was embarrassed by the fact that he had to share a bed with a much younger cousin. Dreaming of his wife one night, he had even taken the young man in his arms:

> It's not good, ah, you know, sleeping in the same bed with a man, a young man. No, it's not in order—he's too young. O.K, with my friend we can [share a bed]. I mean with my age-mate, but that boy—he's just too young. Tony, there are so many things that happen. Like whilst you are sleeping there in bed, you start dreaming. I mean, the way I dream sometimes, I dream loudly. I even talk. So such things. Ah, the other time he told me, "When you were sleeping, you were saying 'Eh, my madam, I press here?'" You see, as if I'm doing it [having sex] and I was calling my wife's name. I mean, I even held my cousin, imagine! So, he shouted, "Ah, what are you doing?" "Ah, yah—sorry!" The guy's my cousin (laughing)—so you see it's awkward.

Promise spent much of 2002 away from the marital home. He and his wife, Susan, were both in paid employment. Before deductions they each earned a little over 200,000 kwacha. They had agreed that they would consider their incomes as their joint money. Their biggest expense was food. On my first stay in their home, including Promise and his children, the household numbered nineteen in the three-bedroom, rat-infested, house. In addition to Promise, Susan, and their children, there was Promise's widowed sister and her three children, two of Promise's nephews, two of his cousins, and his late sister-in-law's son. Susan, Promise's sister, and the children drew water from a nearby well. Food was cooked on braziers outside at the back of the house. For breakfast, there was usually tea and the bread Susan baked. If the budget could not stretch to flour, then the family ate cassava. For lunch they often had fish and *nshima*. In the evening they would eat vegetables and *nshima*. The pressure Promise experienced at home was exacerbated by his desire to assist his mother. He recognized that, "as a man," he was "supposed to provide." The first-born in his family, Promise looked forward to a future when the burden of paying for some of his siblings' education would be lifted as they completed their studies. He concentrated on their education in the hope not that they would assist him in turn but rather that they should at least be independent. He was following his father's example. "In a way (laughing), I am just trying to get rid of my brothers and sisters," he commented. Promise estimated that, since his marriage, he had had about twenty sexual partners. Like many other men in this study, he insisted that having sex with other women in no way implied that he did not love his wife, as the following exchange demonstrates:

> TONY: Would you say you love your wife?
> PROMISE: I do. I do.
> TONY: How do you know that?
> PROMISE: Actions. Actions I do to her, because when she is out [absent from home]—ok, there are times when we are together, ok, we still, ok, we quarrel and what-have-you. But when she is away, as she is now, I always think of her. Yes.

In the year prior to the first of our 2002 interviews, he had had sex with four women, all of whom knew he was a married man with several children. Promise's relationship with one of the women had lasted for some years. Despite her protestations, Promise had "resisted going 'live'" (having unprotected sex), aware as he was that the wife of one of her former partners had recently died of AIDS. Two of the women had already had a sexual relationship with him at earlier points in their lives. According to Promise, one of these women, Lillian, now in her early thirties and childless, complained bitterly when he tried to use a condom, telling him that they had known each other already for years. Promise doubted her claims that there were no other men in her life. Besides, he knew she wanted a child. He had explained to Lillian that he was unprepared to support any child she might have. (Indeed, he was not giving any regular financial support for the children he had fathered before his marriage.) However, she argued that she was ready to support a child on her own. The other woman, Doreen, was the mother of his oldest child. She had not married, nor did she have any other children. He had resolved not to have unprotected sex with her. However, on the several occasions when the condom had burst, Promise told me, "I continued until I had finished because I was drunk." On one visit to see the child, Promise and Doreen went to drink beer. Promise knew that when he was drunk he became "loose." He explained that in their drunken state Doreen had used "sweet talk" and persuaded him to have "three rounds" of unprotected sex: "Her way of talking persuaded me—[saying], 'I don't have anybody.' I told her I was married, but she argued with me: 'If you had married me, I would be the senior wife. You have a child with me! I was the first one to have a child, so I would be the first wife.'" Unlike his school contemporaries, Promise insisted that he did not give his long-term partners money or presents. Indeed, Doreen always roasted a chicken for him to take on his journey and provided transport money. He explained to me that he had begun a relationship with another woman with the encouragement of his best friend, Mwanza, who, within a year, would die of AIDS. One of Mwanza's girlfriends had a woman friend who used to accompany her. In Promise's account, he felt he had been "forced to have sex with her," anxious about what she might think of him if he did not. He thought that there was little trust between men and women, husbands and wives where sex was concerned. Wives did not trust husbands because men tended to have more sexual partners than women. In his judgment it was because men were unable to control their sexual desire. He spoke about friends from his church and elsewhere who were unfaithful to their wives. Promise was well aware that his wife, Susan, did not trust him, though she rarely expressed her suspicions directly. He had only recently broken up with a girlfriend close to home when he discovered she was also having sex with a married policeman. Promise said he was becoming more concerned about the risk of contracting the HIV virus. He was fairly sure that his wife had been aware of the relationship. Following the unprotected sex with Doreen, he said he spent almost a week worrying about AIDS: "I was expecting that this disease could be seen as early as that!" However, he came to the conclusion that it was "better to forget." When he returned home, he immediately resumed having unprotected sex with his wife, though he was aware that she rightly suspected that he had another girlfriend and that he was in the process of trying to establish a relationship with another woman in a nearby town. Susan did not accuse him directly, Promised explained, in ambiguous terms:

> Now the problem with my wife is that when she suspects something, or someone tells her something about a lady somewhere, she cannot come to me directly and say, "This and this." What she wants is to catch me red-handed so that I will not be able to refuse [deny it]. (Laughing.) That's the only goodness. She won't say anything, no. She'll just be looking at you.

Susan knew that Promise's drinking was likely to lead him into relationships with other women. Promise observed: "Over ladies, well, she never usually complains because I have never done it in her presence.... She has heard of me having ladies during our life together, two or three times. She knows it's true, I am a man. I can go out with [have sex with] ladies, yes." Susan set down certain conditions. When Promise came home late, he should not talk to her. The following day, they would be "on good terms." But if Promise failed to keep to their agreement, then she would complain of a headache and refuse to speak to him. Promise did his best to keep to their understanding. They shared the same bedroom, but when he came home late they slept in separate beds.

At one point they quarreled; she intercepted a letter from a woman who appeared eager to establish a relationship with him. Susan's anger soon subsided. Promise discussed their argument in which they spoke about the threat of AIDS without actually naming it:

> She didn't stay angry. I told her the truth: "I talked to her, but I never did anything to her." "No, while you are away, you can do these things. But I know a number of people where you are and they will come and tell me the truth." "It's true. They will come and tell you. But still they may not tell you all the truth. I sleep alone! I am telling you the truth. But if I wanted to, well, I can bring a lady at any awkward hour and others cannot see her! But I don't do that. Yes, I can do it but, now, I also look at you. I look at the children. If I die, you die, who is going to look after these small kids? It's better if we died after this last child has grown up. Also I want a better future for us. Look at the way we are suffering now. No, I want a better future for us and for our children." So she got my words. [She accepted what I was saying.]

After this quarrel, in Promise's estimation, their relationship improved. When they were separated Promise would tell me of the terms of endearment she would use when speaking to him on the phone. During stays in their home, I saw the affection Susan and Promise had for one another. When I asked Promise whether he thought of protecting his wife from the possibility of HIV infection, he questioned how that would be possible:

> Ah, look, there is a problem. There is a problem in marriage if you decide to use a condom. The wife will not trust you. She will suspect. Why? Why are you using a condom? Unless, maybe, you told her, "I've met a lady." And, well, I don't think she would accept you to meet her [have sex with her] even using a condom. No! And then, if you said, "I am not sure [whether I am HIV-positive]," now, for how long are you going to continue using a condom? But, ok, with other ladies you are supposed to use them.

While Promise trusted Susan in sexual matters, he acknowledged that he had "misbehaved" and had given his wife cause not to trust him. Even during her first pregnancy, Promise had started a relationship with another woman. Some years later, Susan physically attacked Promise because of his behavior with another woman. One night one of Promise's regular drinking partners had gone to his home to tell his wife that he was at a bar with a "dead girl" [a woman suspected of suffering from AIDS] and escorted her to the bar. When Susan entered the bar, the woman who had previously had a relationship with Promise ran away. Without a word, Susan proceeded to slap Promise around the head. Then she got hold of his shirt and tried to pull him out of the bar. He explained, indeed boasted to me that, though he and his wife quarreled from time to time, in twelve years of marriage he had never struck Susan. Promise accompanied her home, where he turned the tables against her, pointing out the impropriety of her walking with a man at night. Friends and neighbors intervened to reconcile the couple. Susan often looked sad and became withdrawn when she thought Promise was seeing other women. She preferred not to speak directly of her concerns about his extramarital relationships. On the rare occasions that she challenged Promise, he followed the advice given to him in marriage instruction and denied everything.

Toward the end of 2002, Promise had sexual intercourse on several occasions with Justina, the mother of his second child born before his marriage to Susan. They went drinking together. Justina told him that she was still waiting for him to marry her. She was angry with him for failing to support her and their child. Promise bought the child shoes and gave Justina some money. Whenever they met, they had sex. Promise said the sex was his decision, "though in a way she was giving herself." In the first "round" Promise had used a condom, partly because of the risk of HIV/AIDS but mainly, he explained, because he did not want to make her pregnant again:

> But then, the second round, she complained, saying "Do you think I am sick? Is that why you want to use a condom?" And, to say the truth, I was drunk. I just went out with her live [without a condom]. You see, she complained. She said, "I've never used a condom since I was born. If somebody uses a condom, then they think I am sick." I said, "No, I don't think that you are sick. You are my wife!" "Are you going to marry me?" "Yes, I'll marry you. I'll marry you." (Laughing.) "Then, if you are going to marry me, then, why using a condom?" In a way I was weak. I accepted. But I wasn't that drunk. I would say, well, it was just negligence. It was not just because of beer that I went live, no, because I knew what I was doing, you see. I knew what I was doing. It was just my weakness. I had only one condom. But my intention was just to have one round. But later, when it was about dawn, we started chatting. I felt sex quite ok but I tried to resist. I asked her, "Is it possible that I can go without a condom?" Well, at first she resisted. I mean she pretended that she didn't want to have sex without a condom. She was saying, "Ah, I wouldn't know if you are sick." So me, I said, "Also me, I suspect that you are sick!" We were accusing each other. That's how we ended up having sex without a condom.

When Hambayi and his first wife, Rebecca, started living together she was not pregnant. Their first child was born the following year. Rebecca died three years later shortly after the birth of their second child. Hambayi had just lost his job because of his drunkenness at work and had returned to his father's village where he had become an untrained teacher. When Rebecca fell sick, he took her to the hospital twelve miles from their home. The following day his brother-in-law came to tell him that his wife was dead. According to the hospital the cause of death was malaria aggravated by anemia. Hambayi soon married again. By 2002, he and his second wife, Agatha, had four surviving children. Their first children, twins, had died soon after birth and the child that followed had severe learning difficulties. Hambayi was the sole money-earner in the household in 2002. Agatha had previously sold vegetables at a local market, but Hambayi had told her to stop work and "rest at home." He brought his salary home and gave it to his wife; it was usually around 300,000 kwacha (about U.S. $70) a month. Agatha counted out the money in his presence. He then took what he wanted for his own needs; she kept the rest of the money on a plate in their bedroom. She had to manage the remaining money until the next payday. Hambayi would "beg" beer money from her from time to time in the course of the month. Sometimes, if he seemed low, she would, on her own initiative, give him money for beer. They rented one large room in a shanty compound near Hambayi's workplace. The room was divided into two by lengths of cloth that created a screen between the couple's "bedroom" and the "living room." Their children slept on the floor of the living area together with Hambayi's teenage nephew whom he was also supporting. There was no electricity or piped water in the building. Hambayi resented paying for water from the nearby standpipe. He suspected that most of the money that residents paid for water was stolen by the local party officials who controlled the supply. The family shared a pit latrine with their neighbors. The door of the latrine had a sign that had been removed from the five-star Intercontinental hotel in the city center. The area had numerous bars and shebeens from which music blared out both night and day. At most bars women were available for sex; the prevailing rates were similar to those found in Sampa's compound, that is, 10,000 kwacha for one "round" of sex with a condom and 20,000 kwacha without a condom.

Agatha was seventeen when they married. She had recently failed her grade nine exam and was living at her parents' village when Hambayi sent a small boy with a note that contained a proposal of marriage. Though she had only seen him at the local grinding mill, it did not take her long to accept. Agatha described the roles of husband and wife:

> When a woman gets married she is supposed to look after the home and her husband. She must iron his clothes and heat the water for him to bathe. The man must look after his wife because he is like the father to the woman. Whatever is needed at home, the man must provide. The man should never appear dirty. He also needs to eat. When he comes back from work, the man must find food has been prepared for him. Once the woman has welcomed the husband back home, she has to bring water to the bathroom. After his bath, he has to be given food.

Agatha usually disciplined the young children but she said she needed her husband to discipline the older boys. Hambayi had agreed; she should discipline the girls and he would discipline the boys. She said she had had no say in planning the births of their children. Hambayi was against using condoms. He said God was the one who gave children. It was God's decision. After the birth of their fourth surviving child, Agatha refused to have any more children. With her husband's agreement, she started to receive contraceptive injections at a local clinic. However, within eighteen months, Agatha gave birth to a baby boy. Hambayi and Agatha appeared genuinely fond of one another. While Hambayi said that he trusted his wife, Agatha was anxious about her husband's behavior. She did not trust him, though she had never told him this directly and she had no evidence to confirm her suspicions about his sexual infidelities:

> From the bottom of my heart, I wouldn't trust a man. Men move around. Us women can look after ourselves, but men are fond of admiring women. That is how they are made. Men are a problem. My husband might appear humble and good at home but when he goes away he may be relating to other women. You can be scared. It is important to be courageous.

In fact, Hambayi gave no indication that he was engaged in extramarital sex, though he spoke to me about the "temptations" offered by women at local bars, especially when he was drunk. Hambayi got angry if Agatha did not tell him where she was going when she left the household. He was unhappy about the Bible study sessions she attended at night, suspecting that she was seeing other men. Though she felt shy, she asked him for sex when she wanted it. She thought that all wives should be encouraged to express their sexual desires and preferences. Sometimes she felt too tired to have sex with her husband and did not know how to deal with Hambayi's anger when his desire was denied. (Alternatives such as oral sex were not an option for Hambayi who described such activity as "inhuman.") Agatha had discussed the problem of her husband's sexual demands with women at her Baptist church, but they had advised her that it was her duty to "submit" to her husband's wishes. Though she and her husband quarreled from time to time, they had not contemplated divorce. Agatha thought divorces were caused by wives' lack of respect for their husbands and by men's extramarital affairs, commenting, "If one of these women outside marriage does things [performs sex] in a more satisfactory manner than the wife at home, then the man may want a divorce."

Henry and Pamela enjoyed a much more companionable marriage than many of their contemporaries. Henry had managed to buy a townhouse and he drove a company car. Though he earned more than 2.5 million kwacha (about U.S. $550) a month, he found it difficult to meet all his expenses, especially electricity, water, and school fees. The couple told relatives that they could not support long-stay visitors in their home. Henry drank heavily, but did not consider cutting back on alcohol because, he explained, it was his only form of relaxation. He provided Pamela with capital to start her own cross-border trade in brandy from Zimbabwe. She had free use of the profits. Pamela, who had completed grade twelve, had been secluded when she began to menstruate, though she explained that she was now unable to recall in any detail the content of the lessons. Still, she appreciated them, commenting, "The lessons have helped me to look after my husband, how to give him respect and how to care for him." She wanted her daughters to receive similar instruction because, she explained, growing up in towns, girls did not know the traditions of their people. When her oldest daughter first menstruated, Pamela called one of the women elders in her church who came to give her some medicine—roots soaked in water. Pamela considered that the roles of husband and wife should complement one another. Her husband was "the breadwinner of the house" and her duty was to take care of him, their children, and their home. The couple attended social functions together. However, Henry's excessive drinking caused difficulties in the marriage.[5] In drunken rages he would beat Pamela. While Henry acknowledged his actions to me, she was not prepared to discuss his behavior. Still, she described the influence she believed she had over him: "Nobody, even his own mother has control over him. Everyone looks at me to control him." Pamela agreed with the saying that a man's wife was his mother. She recalled her grandparents' marriage and drew lessons of care from it:

> In a way I think marriage is the same as it was before, only that we are living in a modern world. When I was young I saw my grandmother prepare groundnuts for my grandfather. She would also cut my grandfather's nails. I remember laughing at her. I would ask her why she was doing all that for my grandfather. When I grew up, I recalled these things and I now see that marriage for a woman is all about that—taking care of the husband.

When, soon after their wedding, Henry was separated from his wife because of work, he began a relationship with a younger, unmarried woman whom he had known prior to his marriage. They had not had sex before; within a short while she became pregnant. For some time, Henry was able to keep knowledge of his affair and of the existence of the baby from Pamela. When she found out, Henry promised to end the relationship, but provided financial support for the child. Pamela refused to allow him to bring the child into their home. In the short term, Henry explained, the way his wife had reacted had endeared her even more to him. However, he was distressed that he could not bring his child under his roof. He speculated that, whether Pamela liked it or not, there would come a time when his child would insist on her right to visit him.

Henry had several extramarital partners. In 2002 he had two long-term relationships with unmarried women in different towns. With one girlfriend he had unprotected sex, but with the other he used condoms at times because of his partner's determination not to become pregnant. Pamela had her suspicions about her husband's behavior. Henry thought he should do all he could to hide his relationships with other women from his wife:

> If you have got some indiscretions somewhere, it's better you keep them in a very, very strong safe. You don't let them out so that you don't lose. What's best is not for you to be found out. You die with your secrets. Me, I trust no one—not my wife, not my mother, no one. I don't trust anyone. Maybe, it's because we are all human. We have our own failures, our own weaknesses.

Mutinta and Mutale, both university graduates, enjoyed a companionable marriage in which there appeared to be a good deal of give and take. Their combined monthly income was in excess of 7 million kwacha. They lived in a large house that Mutinta had had built according to his own design. The family had access to two vehicles, one a company car provided for Mutinta, and the other a family saloon that Mutale usually drove. Mutinta recognized that his marriage was very different from that of many of his school contemporaries. He thought that Zambian culture taught people never to trust anyone. However, he said he had complete trust in his wife and his parents; he trusted most of his siblings, at least to a certain extent. He did not engage in extramarital sex. He preferred staying at home to drinking in bars with male friends. At social functions Mutinta realized that he made his work colleagues uncomfortable as he insisted on bringing his wife while they left their wives at home and came with their girlfriends. In his judgment: "It's a sort of achievement for a married man to have a girlfriend. I don't discuss this with them. Perhaps they do this out of lust."

At her first menstruation, Mutale had received some brief lessons about cleanliness and admonitions against having sex with boys. The week before her kitchen party,[6] a group of women elders came to give her marriage instruction. She found some of this helpful—how to be accommodating, unselfish, and tolerant—though she was not prepared to accept every aspect of the teaching she received. She recalled: "There was also the traditional stuff that the wife must be submissive to her husband, but I think we have to meet halfway. This is what prevails in our marriage. My husband knows that I have a say." Mutale painted a picture of equality in her marriage, a portrait echoed independently by her husband. She considered her own sexual desires of equal importance to those of her husband. Both of them should be willing to compromise and only have sex when they both wanted. On the number of children they might have, Mutinta said that that was entirely his wife's decision. Mutale concurred, "I am not under any pressure. If I really wanted, I would have another child." Though Mutinta saw himself as the "provider" in the home, he recognized this was a role that society demanded of him. There had been times when his wife had earned more than him, but this had not caused any problem between them. They jointly agreed the household budget. Mutale observed: "Since we both work, sometimes I spend my salary on my own things. He doesn't have a problem with that. He knows how much I earn and he doesn't dictate. He ensures that the bills are paid. He pays for most of the things, but I do what I can."

Mutinta assisted with childcare and household chores, and explained that he "felt bad" if his wife did something for him that he was perfectly capable of doing for himself. Mutale spoke about how they assisted one another: "When my husband is committed, I will take the car to the garage and when I am busy he will ensure that the children's homework is done." Generalizing from her own experience and that of her university contemporaries, Mutale argued that the position of women in Zambia had improved: "A lot has changed between when our parents married and our marriage. In those days the woman had no say. Now the woman can make decisions. Women are more independent, more educated and more enlightened."

In Mutinta's opinion, many women wrongly married "out of lust" and because they were desirous of wealth. Their desire for security caused them to compromise and to accept their husbands' extramarital relationships. This acquiescence led to their husbands abusing them. Mutale offered very similar observations: "People marry for the wrong reasons. They don't marry for love. They don't marry for companionship. They look for material or financial gain. And also people marry people they can't relate to."

Chalwe and his wife, Anne, were also university graduates and they were both employed in graduate-entry jobs. When he was young, Chalwe explained that he had doubted that he would ever marry: "I was even contemplating priesthood. I've always been a very shy person. I am very docile and very timid. I fear girls a lot." Chalwe and Anne had a white wedding. They married in a Catholic church, though Anne was a Baptist. Chalwe tried to "balance" by attending services in both churches from time to time. He regretted that, unlike his wife, he had received no traditional teaching because of a mix-up in the wedding arrangements; he was sure that some of this teaching would have been beneficial:

> My wife went through quite a rigorous session with the old women and she feels that if I had gone through some teaching, then some of the small problems that we've had would never have occurred. I think the traditional aspects of our sexuality have been there since time immemorial and so it is important for us to keep them.

Anne explained that she had been taught that she must show her husband respect at all times. She must make sure that he was clean and that his clothes were washed and ironed. She was also instructed that she should always be ready to satisfy his sexual needs. From what she was taught and from what she had later learnt, she considered it her right to expect to be sexually satisfied. Before marriage, Anne received both church and "traditional" instruction:

> I have found the lessons I learnt, especially the traditional teaching, helpful in marriage. I was taught how to look after my husband, to look after his body, how to respect him and to keep myself clean at all times. I remember when I was made to grab a stone from the mouth of one of my instructors, using only my mouth. It was about holding on to my husband when somebody else is trying to snatch him away from me. I was taught I must endure in marriage.

Anne, like Mutale, considered that the position of a wife had improved for women of her generation—especially those who were university graduates living in town, though there were aspects of the "traditional" that she wished to maintain, judging that Western influence was harmful. "We are throwing away tradition," she observed, "and copying the Western culture that we don't really understand." On the negative side, in the past, and still in many villages, women were left to do most of the work, while men waited to be served. Anne's expectations appeared to be a blend of the "traditional" and the "modern" when it came to her own marriage:

> The man is expected to financially support the home and in terms of decisions he has the last say. He is supposed to clean the physical surroundings. If he doesn't mind, he can also do some house cleaning, especially when there are children in the marriage. The woman has to

take care of the family, making sure that everybody is comfortable and fed.

Chalwe and Anne put their monthly incomes, each of about 2 million kwacha, together and jointly agreed the household budget. Chalwe explained that in the first years of his marriage, he had quarreled with his wife over money. She had insisted on knowing exactly what he earned. Even though the Catholic marriage instruction had stressed the importance of being open to one's partner, Chalwe said he had come under the influence of his male friends who, he explained, had told him, "You cannot give your income to your madam [wife]." In the face of his wife's repeated challenges he had relented, though he still had his reservations: "She told me, 'When you get your pay, you must bring it to me! You are supposed to bring everything here!' But she's earning a salary, and I'm not supposed to ask her anything. I find it strange that we don't discuss [what to do with] *her* salary." Chalwe thought it was very important to have children. He and Anne had two. Having no children would "send the wrong signal" and a man would not feel complete. If he wanted another child he would have to discuss this with his wife, but three children would be the absolute limit because of expensive town life. Anne explained that their two children were planned. She and her husband had agreed that she would use the pill, though they had occasionally used condoms. She said that they would both have to agree if they were to have another child. Anne, like Pamela, did not wish to discuss any doubts she might have about her husband's sexual fidelity to her. She explained that she *chose* to trust Chalwe, "I trust him. When there is no trust, then it becomes difficult. You can't trust only 90% because the 10% lack of trust will destroy the rest." Chalwe pondered the question of trust for some time before commenting, "From my experience, I don't think that there is anyone that I trust. No, no one."

Conclusion

I witnessed the degree of care and comfort that wives of former students normally gave their husbands. Men and women commonly observed, "Your wife is your mother." Wives prepared water for men to bathe—indeed they often bathed them; they cooked or, where there were domestic workers, supervised the cooking of meals and announced in a respectful posture, either kneeling or seated, when meals were ready.[7] Wives washed or supervised the washing of husbands' clothes, and cleaned or supervised the daily cleaning of homes.

Wives and other female household members spent an extraordinary amount of time and energy each day in sweeping and mopping floors. In receiving personal care and attention from wives and other women, men both acknowledged their need to be taken care of by women and demonstrated their right, as adult men, to such services. Recognizing their dependence, men revealed a degree of ambivalence toward the much-vaunted values of male independence and self-sufficiency inculcated in them from an early age, even though most were determined to show that they retained the upper hand in their marriage. In the domestic domain, however, almost all wives controlled the household budget. In this regard wives were considered trustworthy, better able to budget than their husbands. Household matters, especially decisions about meals, were the concern of women, though some men, especially those who had a car, often went food shopping with their wives.[8] In general, wives in paid employment considered their earnings as their own, to spend as *they* pleased. It was the husband's responsibility to provide for the family's day-to-day needs and to maintain the family home. In men's eyes, as in women's, that was the meaning of marriage. Such expectations in urban marriages have been recorded on the Copperbelt in the 1950s (Epstein 1981: 311) and in Lusaka in the 1980s (Hansen 1996: 120; ibid.: 162). This pressure on men to be "breadwinners" was keenly felt by former students. They became despondent when they perceived that they had "failed" because of low pay or unemployment.

Asserting the right to make all the key decisions in the family and household, many men justified their claim to their "superior" position in marriage by reference to "African tradition" and to Christianity. However, analysis of marriage relations revealed the performance of a range of masculinities among former students; some men acknowledged that there were other ways of being a husband, deferring to their wives, assisting in household chores and childcare, even when they recognized that others might read this as "weakness." Here at least some degree of equitable relationships was made possible, especially where such matters as the number of children a couple might have was mutually agreed between husband and wife, or, in exceptional instances, was decided by a wife alone.

Some men, such as Mutinta, Paul, Peter, and Joshua, abstained from extramarital sex. Many men felt the pressure of their peers— real or imagined—to show that they were "real men," capable of "controlling" their wives. For most men, this impression management entailed engaging in extramarital affairs. In addition, almost all former students described sex as an urgent need that had to be repeatedly satisfied. Many men appeared to surrender their claims of self-sufficiency, especially when under the influence of alcohol. "Self-control" in sexual matters did not appear to be a value held by many men. Women concurred that this was how men were "made," different from women who were able to go for weeks and even months without sex. If work or family matters separated husband and wife for more than a few days, the expectation was that men would seek "relief" elsewhere. Most wives feared that when their husbands were not sexually satisfied at home—and even when they were—they would seek other partners. However, contrary to the marriage instruction they had received from *banacimbusa*, wives claimed their right to sexual satisfaction from their husbands and some sought this satisfaction elsewhere. Most wives were not "in denial" about their husbands' extramarital activities.[9] While they feared HIV risk, they did not confront their husbands and often appeared both unable and unwilling to seek a divorce. Their role was to endure, whatever the costs.[10] Despite wives' fears, there was evidence of real affection and friendship between many husbands and wives. While I heard numerous echoes of the distrust reported by earlier ethnographers of urban marriage in Zambia, I rarely encountered, for example, the ferocious misogyny reported among miners by Ferguson.

While observing, "Men are a problem" and "Men are difficult," women commonly noted of their husbands, "Men are children." As far as wives were concerned, men's "childishness" was most clearly—and most dangerously—revealed in their pursuit of extramarital, unprotected, sex. Men explained to me that their extramarital relationships did not mean that they did not love their wives. Most insisted that their extramarital affairs were a completely separate matter and appeared genuinely surprised when I tried to discuss the potential dangers that their unprotected extramarital sex posed for their wives. They commonly met my inquiries with comments such as "This has got nothing to do with my wife" and "Why are you bringing my wife into this?" Some former students suggested to me that their extramarital sex was a consequence of a distinct "African sexuality." I explore this contention, together with men's sexual preferences and understandings of forms of sexual activity, in chapter 6.

6

SEXUALITY AS A SITE OF DIFFERENCE

The HIV/AIDS pandemic in Zambia is driven, at least in part, by particular expressions of heterosexual masculinities. This chapter describes aspects of former students' sexual repertoire. My purpose is to investigate what "sex" meant for these men and to throw light on their sexual conduct, fully aware as they were of the extent of the pandemic. The majority of former students regarded sexual activity as a site of difference between "Europeans" (whites) and "Africans" (blacks); in conversations and interviews they produced essentialized and opposed "African" and "European" sexualities, not unlike some "European" commentators.[1] All the men interviewed had had sexual intercourse only with black Africans. In general, their ideas about "European" sexuality were gleaned from television, films, "blue movie" videos, and pornographic novels. The category "African" was linked to the notion of "tradition," while "European" was associated with, and indeed considered synonymous with, the term "modern." Moral evaluations of the two supposedly distinct sexualities were contested. Some men presented a self-critical view of "African sexuality," portraying African males as unable to control their sexual desires.[2] However, while European men might be supposed to have greater self-control, there was much debate as to whether their "modern" sexuality was evidence of an advanced culture or of immorality.[3] Some men claimed the moral high ground for Africa. In their view Africans treated sex as sacred, unlike "loose Europeans." They said Africans treated sexual matters in a "respectable way," acting with public restraint. What was said to be the "European" propensity of men and women to kiss and hug in public, described as taboo behavior in Zambia, was understood to signal the desire for, or the existence of, a sexual relationship.[4] Darius commented, "Europeans treat sex like eating.

They talk about sex as though they were talking about food. But for us to talk like that is taboo."[5] Edmund observed, "I think the African culture puts a lot of value on sex and fecundity. Here sex is a little sacred but there in Europe it can be done openly. The way people treat each other in public, like kissing, hugging—we never approve that here."

Former students emphasized that for "African" men and women penetration was the defining feature of sex. Anything short of penetration was not considered to be "sex." Malama summed up some of the supposed differences between the "races" as follows:

> In Africa, the way sex is handled is in such a way that we believe so much in the penetration of a man into a woman. It's then that the sexual act is completed. In Africa we don't believe that you need to arouse the woman's sexual appetite, no, but in Europe they believe in doing that before they have sexual intercourse. And even the way they have sexual intercourse, it is different from the way we have sex here. I mean here we believe in the woman lying down and then you climb on top of her—things like that.

The village was the reference point for the space of authentic African sex, the arena where male "sexual strength" was most forcefully expressed. Many former students argued that African men surpassed European men in this strength. All men identified extended foreplay prior to vaginal penetration as a distinguishing feature of European sexuality. Those who evaluated European sexuality positively strove to imitate it, at least in this regard, though few enjoyed "wet sex" (see later).[6] Darius, explaining that he had adopted "the Western style," kissing and fondling his wife prior to penetration, commented, "Traditionally there is nothing like caressing and kissing. As the man, you just command that you want to have sex." Village men, according to Darius, were "a stronger breed" who did not believe that a woman's "sexual appetite" should first be aroused: "Some villagers have confessed to me that they have thirteen children but they have never played with [fondled] the wife. They have never even kissed. Meanwhile they have thirteen children. For me I have to kiss and touch her here and there. For them it is straight in."

Some former students considered that it all came down to a question of education, by which they meant access to "modern" Western education. They regretted, "Africans have not learned much about how to do these things." For "uneducated villagers" there was "no time-wasting in sex," where men "jump like bulls."

Many men felt under pressure to claim sexual knowledge and experience. Sexual partners should be convinced of their expertise by their performance during intercourse. Wives and girlfriends should feel sexually satisfied. At bars and beer parties, men should be able to speak authoritatively with other men on sexual matters. In producing narratives of their sexual exploits, they should demonstrate that they were good at being men (see Herzfeld 1985). As in their schooldays, they felt the requirement to compose persuasive accounts of their conquests. Dominic considered this pressure to be particularly strong in Africa:

> It's funny the way we Africans behave. I am saying that because, you see, if you haven't had sex in your life, well, you are not regarded as a man. You are not a man in Africa. Because one of the qualifications—I don't know whether I should call it a certificate—(laughing) well, for you to be considered as part of the group, the group of men, the group of adults, you need to experience sex. When you go to certain places, well, you find that men are discussing; they are discussing sex. Imagine you are just there; you are quiet! You are not contributing! So the men in the group will say, "Hey, are you okay, my friend?" I mean when you are there and there are these discussions, well, you have to contribute something: "No, me, I did this! I remember once I did this—what-and-what." So when you do that, that puts you now in a different category. Now you are in the category of adults. Well, even me, I will be—I am a little bit traditional—you know, women, when you go deep, when you go very deep in an African society, African women don't like men who have had no experience in terms of sex. They feel you are wasting their time. The man should be active. He should know what to do. In our case, us Africans, well, we regard women, as, well, they should be passive, when it comes to sex. I don't know how you look at it, Tony, but the man is supposed to initiate sex. A woman cannot initiate sex, no!

Most men had experimented with various herbs and roots in their youth and many continued to use them in adult life to maintain or improve their sexual performance.[7] The most common substance, "gunpowder," was sold by women in markets and at bars. Some men were opposed to the use of such *muti* for a range of reasons. Seventh Day Adventists and Born Agains rejected medicine made from "roots" as they suspected their preparation involved "traditional," that is unchristian, mystical practices. A few men doubted their efficacy. They had noticed no improvement in their performance. Others were very impressed. Medicine from "outside" (abroad) was attributed greater efficacy. Darius spoke excitedly of medicine he knew as

Ufu, a powder that he would put in a drink. He first obtained it on a trip to Zimbabwe, not long after he left school:

> It really works. I wanted to have more sex. With a usual partner I normally only do it twice a night. But with *Ufu* I did it six times with my girlfriend! She noticed the difference and I confessed that it was because of the *Ufu*. That first time I used it for two months. I got tired! It made me stronger. I don't know whether the sperm was coming out or not, but I didn't feel it was coming out as I normally do. What happened was my erection remained or came back quicker! I think my girlfriend enjoyed it too. I should think so because we mostly leave our friends [sexual partners] hanging [not sexually satisfied] if we tire out after two rounds. I hate it when I have ejaculated and feel I have finished but my friend still wants more. It is best I make her satisfied and I satisfy myself.

When men like Sampa and Malama were engaged in extramarital affairs, they valued aphrodisiacs all the more, convinced they helped to guard them from a wife's suspicions. Malama observed: "You find that you need to be in form. I mean you need to be energetic so that you perform well. And then, in addition, there is an obligation that you have to perform at home. So to be actually able to do that, well, you have to go for something to help you."

Sampa was cautious about buying powders from women at bars, suspecting that their concoctions were often nothing more than sawdust. He had more faith in other produce:

> I use some green stuff called *kola*, but I don't have any at the moment. It's used by these Senegalese. Now when you eat that—it's some sort of fruit. You are probably aware that these Senegalese are well up in these matters. You eat that fruit. Now maybe one hour later, well, if I meet [have sex with] a lady, ah, it's terrible! It's terrible!

Many men found that some everyday foodstuffs stimulated their sexual appetite and improved their performance. They noted that fresh groundnuts and bitter cassava, in particular, increased the amount of semen they produced.

Tight and Dry Sex

All the men were aware of campaigns warning of the increased risk of HIV transmission in tight and dry sex and did not doubt the biomedical explanations they were given. However, most of those interviewed stressed that tight and dry sex was the most pleasurable way to have intercourse.[8] There was general agreement among older women that a young woman's body should be prepared to maximize the pleasure of her husband-to-be. This guided marriage instruction. Women instructors (*banacimbusa*) encouraged young women to make their vaginas tight and dry to heighten men's pleasure in sex. The instructors obtained herbs that the brides-to-be were instructed to take in their porridge. They advised bathing in cold water when herbs were not available. They noted the greater possibility of bruising for men, though no explicit connection was made to HIV transmission or to the particular risk to women. Older women colluded with men in the fantasy of male power, of masculine conquest. In sexual intercourse, a husband should experience the sense of having conquered his wife; he should feel that through his own manly efforts he has achieved his goal. As one instructor commented, "The man's penis should not enter without difficulty; he should struggle." Wives were expected to have stretched their labia minore prior to marriage.[9] "If the girl does not have extended labia, she will feel shy in marriage," instructors explained during interviews conducted in Lusaka in 2002. They said that such preparation might cause women to become "wet" during intercourse, something disliked by most men, as one *banacimbusa* explained:

> Long labia produce a lot of excretion. They make so much noise during sex that it can be heard from those sleeping in the next room. Men don't like wet vaginas. The penis must feel as if it has been grabbed by something and not whereby it slides in as if it is a train on a rail. When the man touches them [the labia], they should feel nicely thick and when he enters the woman he only feels her sweetness.

Most men said that for the woman to have a dry vagina was "the traditional way." In this regard, "tradition" was more attractive than "modernity." They understood that wives prepared their bodies in this way as "a sign of respect." No man spoke of drying their partners, though this has been reported by other commentators in Zambia. (See Hira et al. 1990.)

Many former students explained that a wet vagina was slippery and uncomfortable and the man might easily withdraw unintentionally. For a man to enjoy intercourse and be satisfied, the woman's vagina should be dry and warm inside. This also helped the man to achieve speedy ejaculation. Former students knew that many women took medicine to make themselves "warm" and to excite any man who came close to them or touched them. The beads that many women wore around their waists were also treated with medicine to stimulate a man's desire and to make him feel "warm and nice" when he was on top of her during sex. The desire to feel the penis in a warm, dry place figures regularly in men's descriptions. It seems to suggest the desire to find a comforting, safe place, perhaps a refuge from a world that was often felt to be uncomfortable and discomforting.

In adulthood, as in his youth, sex for Sampa always felt "nicer" when it was "fast" (when he ejaculated quickly). It was for this reason that he preferred "tight and dry" sex: "When the woman is tight and dry, that's when you really feel the nice friction! Besides, no woman wants to be called '*mugodi*' ('a mine')." However, he had begun to reflect that this kind of sex was "not fair on the woman," because of the pain it might cause them and because of the widely reported increased risk of HIV transmission:

> If the woman is tight, ah, that's very nice. I prefer tight and dry. These days they are saying that it is not advisable because of AIDS: the more the vagina is actually tight, the more you risk something, because of the friction. But, as for me, I believe tight cunts are nice. That's when you really feel something nice—the friction—unlike when it's watery. When it's watery, you don't feel anything. These days women still try to make themselves tight and dry.

Enoch also spoke of his enjoyment of "tight and dry" sex. Assuming his preference was the norm among most men, he commented, "We men want to feel something." Enoch was sure that women liked tight and dry sex. He appeared to assume that I was critical of this practice, as the following interview extract reveals: "Women do enjoy tight and dry sex. I've also heard that women in Europe (laughing)—ah, I'm attacking you now!—women in Europe would rather give birth by Caesarian section rather than spontaneous delivery just to keep the vagina tight."

Darius explained to me his preference for tight and dry sex, though he too recognized that, in drying themselves to please men, women increased the risk of HIV transmission:

> When the thing is not tight and it is wet, you feel you are not with somebody but alone. You really have to have that friction to feel you are with somebody. I think they [women] equally enjoy it dry. They have the same feeling. They feel you are there with them when it is dry and tight. Also it means I can ejaculate faster and go for more rounds. African women even take medicines and, when they are wet, they will excuse themselves so that they can clean themselves—dry themselves up. They feel embarrassed when they come out wet.

Some of those who worked in the health sector were concerned about the potential for abrasions to be caused. Simon felt pity for women who felt they had to dry themselves for men's sexual satisfaction and bemoaned the fact that many men who should know better could not forego some of their sexual pleasure:

> I think women are taught to please men and they are told that that is how men want them to be. So as much as possible they dry themselves for him as much as for themselves. I think in Zambia, mostly, it is about men getting their satisfaction. And then again, there is a lot of ignorance, especially about female sexuality. And maybe even the women themselves sometimes don't understand that either. You know, in Zambia, well the man has had his satisfaction, so that's the end of it and as for them [the women], well, they shouldn't complain about it. They don't complain much. I mean even for myself, it's only through reading and learning biology that I have come to understand things like lag-time, that women come later than men, that men come more quickly. It's something that is never discussed. That's why I mean there is that level of ignorance. For men, for many men, it's just about them coming and that's it. Well, it used to be a problem in the West as well, but now it is something that is recognized.

George and Paul recognized the dangers of tight and dry sex. While this was their preference, they likened such sex to rape.

"Styles" and "Rounds"

Men repeatedly spoke of supposed differences between "African" and "European" women. They referred me to the initiation in which a Zambian woman learnt how to please a man and assumed that such instruction was not given to a European woman. Some of the men's female cousins had offered them detailed accounts of their own initiation when a female instructor "took the part of the man" and climbed on top of them, and of how she had pinched them when they failed to "dance properly." Edmund's Italian fellow worker praised Zambian women's sexual skills: "Zambian Maria is very good. The way she dances in bed, it's like a concrete mixer." Former students judged women from the east of the country to be particularly adept. Sampa was among many men who sang the praises of women from Eastern Province:

> Traditionally, we Blacks, this is the way we are. Black ladies, they prefer making a lot of movements when the man is on top. Also the man, he

is also making some movements. So these ladies from Chipata are very good at that.[10] That's what I prefer. There's supposed to be some proper movement. Proper movement! (Laughing.) The ladies are taught. You know the woman's dancing, it's just exaggerated—the movements of the body—the buttocks—while you are inside her.

Many former students appeared to be quite conservative in their sexual techniques. The childhood idea that the "correct" manner was for the male to lie on top of the female endured. Men repeatedly explained to me that this was the "proper African" position and used the term "climb on top of the woman" as if to emphasize their dominant, powerful position, though they also spoke about being "powerless" immediately after ejaculation. Notions of "respectability" held sway with regard to positions—"styles." A minority of former students reported trying different positions, especially, though not exclusively, in extramarital sex—a consequence, they suggested, of Western influence. European men were said to be ready to "allow" the woman to be on top of the man. Some former students were anxious about having intercourse with the woman "on top." They worried that their semen might not properly enter their partner and that, because of this, the act of sexual intercourse would not be complete. As Darius explained, "I just believe the sperms will come back down. I feel sex is not completed if sperms don't go in." In addition, because some women were "rough," the penis might be injured. Indeed men complained that they found intercourse in this position both painful and exhausting. It was in this position that the few men who used condoms found they were most likely to burst.

Promise, like Darius, had learnt from films how "to enter from behind, on the edge of the bed." For Promise being on top in extramarital sexual intercourse was not particularly important. He had experimented with different positions that he had seen portrayed and noted his partners' enjoyment of the variety:

> With these pornography films we have been watching, ah, we have learnt a number of styles (laughing). And you find these ladies, ah, especially these common ladies, they'd prefer that you do it in a number of styles. Like, for example, they will tell you that they want you to do it backwards—I mean into her vagina but from behind. Then there is this other one called "Scissors" whereby you lie down, both facing one side. She gives you her back, then the lady in front, she lifts one leg, then you enter. Then you form more or less like a scissors. And that's the one now that most of the ladies are preferring. They say that's when they really feel it—when the whole stuff goes in! (Laughing.)

A number of men recognized that not all women were the same in their sexual responses and so "timing" became important if they wished to satisfy their partner. Their comments indicated that during sexual intercourse there was at least some communication between partners. Promise, who had affairs that lasted several years, was aware of the need to satisfy a girlfriend if he wished to "keep" her. He explained that he tried to tailor his sexual performance to what he knew of his partner:

> There are some ladies who would like you to do it as early as possible, but for others, they take time to reach that sensational point. Maybe, you even get tired, "Ah, no, it's too much!" You would release [ejaculate], you would release, but she is still holding on you.... It depends on the lady. If I have stayed with a lady, then I will know the duration in which this lady gets that feeling. So I will have to time. There are times when I am meeting such a lady, well, when I feel like releasing, I withdraw to give her time also to have that feeling. So I withdraw for a while and maybe I just start playing with her, using my hands, my fingers, then I go back in.

A partner's reported sexual satisfaction was evidently a source of reassurance. George was particularly anxious to satisfy his wife. They usually had sex three or four times a week, most frequently over weekends, he explained:

> There are situations when I get satisfied before she does. In trying to satisfy her, I would do it twice, three or even four times. I think it is a problem we have. It rarely happens that both of us get satisfied at the same time. It is very important to satisfy my wife because I know marriages that have broken up because one of the partners could not get sexual satisfaction. She tells me when she is not satisfied.

Men gave different estimates of the desired number of rounds of sex in a session of sexual intercourse and their preferred frequency, which, some noted in intercourse with their wives, had declined with age and years of marriage. Former students recognized that factors that affected their desire and their performance included their own physical condition and energy levels, the sexual partner—whether wife, girlfriend, or stranger— and the stage and length of a relationship, and whether they were paying for sex. In most accounts the greater the number of rounds the greater were the claims of potency.[11] Several men rated themselves "above average in sexual strength," that is capable of more than two or three rounds in one "session." Darius noted differences between sex with his wife and with his extramarital partners, especially new girlfriends. With his wife, he found two rounds at night and a further two in the early morning was his norm. He recognized that his sexual activity was governed by his moods. In a good mood he might have four rounds and try different positions. At other times he might go as long as a week without sexual intercourse, but on average he estimated that he would usually have about fourteen rounds with his wife in a week. As they grew older, some men reevaluated what they considered desirable. While as young men they claimed it was not uncommon for them to have four or five rounds, several had come to consider that two "well-done rounds" in a night were now sufficient.

WITHDRAWAL

Men said withdrawal was a difficult skill to master. It was not a popular method of birth control because it was "not a hundred per cent thing." Men objected, in particular, to the loss of pleasure, "at the most exciting part." Several asked me rhetorically, "What is the point of withdrawing when you are on the point of firing?" Besides, it was not "proper sex." Better not to begin intercourse at all. Many men recalled seeing *coitus interruptus* in pornographic films. They gave it as yet another example of Western influence, even though, unknown to them, it was common practice among at least some of their grandparents' generation.[12] Few men spoke of using withdrawal with their wives, except in "emergencies" such as when a wife had not taken a contraceptive pill. As a technique that requires a considerable degree of communication and cooperation between the partners, the relative infrequency of the use of withdrawal, both within marriage and in extramarital relationships, may indicate the absence of an equitable relationship. (See Schneider and Schneider 1995; Santow 1993.) Besides, the ready availability of various forms of female contraception clearly made withdrawal an unappealing—indeed what they saw as an unnecessary—option for men. It was sometimes attempted with premarital and extramarital partners. However, as Malama commented, "When sex is out of wedlock, you don't go home a proud man if you don't release inside—and, besides, you don't feel that you have had sex." However, competence in withdrawal might also entail a claim to manliness, to being a "real man." In the men's estimation, withdrawal technique required "strength" as much as skill and a high degree of self-control. George remembered his biology teacher, a married Zambian man, in senior school likening sex to the game of football and referring to withdrawal as "shooting wide of the goalmouth." George was against it, mostly because, in his experience, it was easy to make mistakes. Men's technique improved with practice and age, though several noted that, apart from their own denial of pleasure, their partners were not satisfied. Peter was against withdrawal because he considered that the moment of ejaculation was the highest expression of love for his wife. Sampa said it was better to use a condom than to practice withdrawal, though he was against both. He spoke at some length about the loss of pleasure and, as others, likened withdrawal to masturbation—something he did not normally approve of. He had only tried withdrawal once, with his girlfriend Josephine, he explained:

> Ah, that one, Tony. Ah—when you are about to release and then you pull out? No, no, me, I can't [do that]. I mean that's the time (laughing)—that's the time when you feel—that's the best time, the time when you feel really, really nice—No I can't, I can't. (Laughing.) No! That's when you feel very nice. No, no—you pull out then and put it somewhere else? Actually this happened recently with Josephine. The very first time I had direct contact with her. We'd used condoms at the beginning. That was the first time that I went direct. So I was there on top, dancing, dancing, and she said, "When you are about to release, please come out." I said to her, "Okay, no problem." So we started, going, going. Now when she can feel that I am about to—so—the moment I wanted to try that one, she herself, she held me tighter, very tightly, very tightly, so, (laughing) ah, it's very difficult. So me, ah, I've never done that myself. I don't like it but I wanted to try. In my case, I think, once you do that, it's the same as masturbation. It's just as if you forget about a woman and you do it yourself. That's why I don't like the idea. It's difficult for me, I mean, I could have done it, you know, because I was afraid that I could make her pregnant, but she held me tightly. I couldn't pull out. She prevented me.

Sampa then described how Josephine had wept because of his failure to withdraw. They did not attempt this technique again. Not long after this incident, Josephine announced that he had made her pregnant. However, Sampa did not think that she had deliberately prevented him from withdrawing.

ATTITUDES AND EXPERIENCE TOWARDS MASTURBATION IN ADULTHOOD

Almost all the men interviewed reported at least some experience of self-masturbation, at some point in their lives. Two men claimed they had never masturbated. On the whole, attitudes toward solitary masturbation remained unchanged in adult life. The men unanimously said it was unsatisfying when compared to "real sex," that is, vaginal penetration. Many described masturbation as "not natural" and "psychologically damaging." Some condemned the practice outright even though—or perhaps because—they had on occasion "given in to temptation." Drawing upon the Bible to vindicate their condemnation, Born Agains and others argued that masturbation was for "sick people" with "corrupt minds." No one mentioned that women might masturbate themselves. I did not ask specifically about this. George was not Born Again but, like many others, referred me to the Bible: "When somebody gets used to that [masturbation], they do not have feelings to [for] the opposite sex. It is also said that the person can be compared to the one who has been castrated. And when you refer to the Bible, especially the story of creation, that wasn't God's intention."

Peter, who in his youth had tried masturbating but found no pleasure in it, noted that masturbation was strongly discouraged at his Seventh Day Adventist Church. Darius, in his mid-thirties, raised a common objection to solitary self-masturbation:

> You really need to feel the person you are with—unlike when you are alone and feel you are having sex. You need to feel the body of the woman. The pleasure of masturbation is not complete because you need the voice of your friend whispering sweet words to you and that is when you feel you are having sex. The best is not to masturbate because you can't go on masturbating for the rest of your life.

Simon at forty noted the general silence in Zambia around the topic of masturbation, remarking, "I mean most people think a person is mad if they talk about it." He had no religious objections. As he had explained twenty years earlier, however, self-masturbation could never replace penetrative intercourse for him. He recognized the potential benefit of mutual masturbation as an alternative to penetrative sex in efforts to prevent the transmission of the HIV virus, but, like others, he found it difficult to see this as an expression of love. He commented, "Masturbating is different from having sex. What about the human feelings for one another? And there is love. It is a whole complex of things." Even Promise, who had enjoyed youthful masturbation competitions, wondered whether his childhood experience had not had a deleterious effect, causing him in later life to engage in extramarital intercourse. He noted that almost all of the village age-mates he had masturbated with were now dead—most of them, he suspected, from AIDS.

As they had done twenty years previously, many men reported that they had been brought up to understand that any touching of the penis or testicles for pleasure was "taboo." In later life they had overcome their shyness when women handled their genitals; for some it helped to ensure speedy ejaculation. Darius explained: "Me, I used to be shy, but now it is something that pleases me. When I am in the act and she [his wife] plays with my testicles it helps me to ejaculate faster." Several men spoke of being masturbated by their wives and other sexual partners. This masturbation most commonly occurred when wives or other sexual partners were menstruating. Sampa maintained his strong disapproval of self-masturbation. He asked his wife to masturbate him when she was "sick," that is, when she was menstruating:

> I mean, in that situation I tell my wife, "Can you do this rather than I go and look for other women?" Then she does it, we kiss, and that is all. I mean, there it is okay, but not in a situation where she is not even sick [menstruating] and then you tell her to masturbate you. No, that's not in order!

Men acknowledged that they enjoyed being masturbated, though, they stressed, it could never become a satisfying alternative to penetration. At best, it might be enjoyed in foreplay. "Why leave the proper part and go elsewhere?" they repeatedly asked me.

ANAL SEX

Former students unanimously condemned adult heterosexual and homosexual anal sex. Men described it as "abuse," "the worst thing," "evil," "immoral," and "against our African values." The notion of "African sexuality" was once more frequently mobilized, as in the following comment from Malama: "Ah, to me, as an African, it's a taboo. As an African whose beliefs are even African, I don't aspire to that, I don't encourage that and the one who practices that, well, to me, he's not a comrade."

Condemnation was primarily expressed in religious terms. Such behavior, the men maintained, contravened God's law. Only two men condemned anal sex on health and hygiene—rather than moral— grounds. Such sex damaged muscles in the anus, they said, and caused bruising that assisted the spread of HIV. Other former students knew this, but did not mention it as part of their objection. While some had been aware of a number of boys practicing anal sex while at primary boarding school and at St. Antony's, the general opinion was that this was "not serious" as the boys were not yet mature. (There was no suggestion here of a "homosexual" stage in sexual development.) No one told me they had any personal experience of it, and few said they knew any adults who engaged in it. There was general recognition that anal sex was common in all-male prisons. Former students maintained that this occurred because of the absence of women and not because of any genuine sexual attraction between men. They understood these acts as attempts to gain relief from sexual tension from the only available sources.

Several former students noted that, given the strength of feeling against anal sex among Zambians, it was a practice that any man who engaged in it, either as inserter or insertee, would need to hide.[13] Speaking of heterosexual anal sex, Promise observed:

> Well, that one, personally I've never experienced it. Ah, no, it's a taboo. (Laughing.) If you happened to tell someone you did that, they'd even laugh at you. They would think maybe—ah, here in Zambia, they would think of many things![14] Why? Why leave the actual part to go and look somewhere else? (Laughing.) Imagine! (Laughing.) No, no, you cannot even disclose it to your friend, no, if you happen to do it! I mean it would be considered abnormal. And I don't think—ah, no, even the lady cannot accept it. No! No!

Oral Sex[15]

As adults, former students considered oral sex a European practice that, with modernity, some Zambians were taking up. "Things are changing fast," I was repeatedly told. Many men had seen it portrayed in pornographic videos and were adamant that this practice was "taboo traditionally." Again the village became a synonym for tradition. A common remark was "Having grown up in the village, we do not try such things." Critics also invoked God's plan of creation; oral sex was "against the Bible," "abnormal," "not fit for human beings," and "insane." God had fashioned each body part for its particular function. A few men noted that while it was not explicitly forbidden in the Bible, and therefore permissible, it held no appeal for them. George spoke of his strong disapproval of oral sex. He saw it as a threat to the order of nature; for him such sexual activity was "out of place":

> I have never tried oral sex but I have seen that in movies—pornographic videos—and I feel that it is wrong. It is wrong because everything has its own place. In the home kitchen utensils are supposed to

be in the kitchen. They cannot be kept in the toilet. Or you can't put toilet paper in the kitchen or the sitting room. God, from the time he created us, knew where things belonged. I am not in favor of someone using things wrongly.

Oral sex was available from "prostitutes" at nightclubs and bars in Lusaka and on the Copperbelt. In 2002, the price with a condom was between 10,000 and 15,000 kwacha and 30,000 kwacha without a condom. Perhaps because it was often associated with "prostitutes," who, men assured me, enjoyed this kind of sex, in our initial discussions only a few men spoke about engaging in it. They did not wish to be associated with what might be judged disreputable activity. However, over the course of a number of interviews, as some of the men appeared to become more comfortable speaking about their sexual experience, they acknowledged that fellatio was pleasurable. While for them it could not replace penetration, they enjoyed fellatio in foreplay and it might at times be an alternative source of "release" when circumstances prevented men from performing vaginal penetration. There were very few reported instances of cunnilingus and these seemed to be only with wives. Many men thought, unlike fellatio, cunnilingus was unhygienic, a "dirty" activity.

Several men said that they had been introduced to fellatio by either a girlfriend or their wife. Women, apparently, had again become men's teachers in erotic pleasure. Men seemed to want to make women responsible for beginning such activity. However, women's reported initiative appears to be another instance where women did not always take a passive role, though men could, of course, interpret women's role in fellatio as passive. Darius told me that he enjoyed oral sex when he was "sexually high": "The first time my wife did it on her own [of her own volition]. After that I ask her when I want it. She swallows my sperm." Some men reported that women complained that this practice–like using a condom in vaginal penetration—was bad because it was "wasting semen."[16]

Sampa requested oral sex when his wife, Ruth, refused him penetrative sex during her menstruation. In one of Ruth's absences, when he was sick in bed with TB, he refused the offer of fellatio from one of his girlfriends who regularly came to visit him. The consequence of semen loss, and hence the loss of physical strength, was uppermost in his mind. He explained to me, he did not want to lose the proteins and hence the energy he needed to recuperate:

> So, you know, we were in bed, she started kissing me. She wanted to suck me, but I refused. I didn't have the power to perform.... That's

why she said, "Can I suck you?" So I said, "No, don't, please." I needed my proteins.... You see, Tony, well, the way I feel right now—You know, I can't hide from you—the way I am feeling at the moment, especially as I am not taking any alcohol, I feel I am really a hundred percent okay. As a result you'll find, well, ok, it's like now I need a lady. So as of now, I am finding it very difficult to sleep like this [without sex]. I refused because of energy. And also because if she sucked me, then I could have ended up now doing the real thing. She could have sucked me; then, in the next round I do it with her. I mean, she herself, while sucking, she could have felt sex. She was then going to force me now to do it.

At other times, Sampa spoke of oral sex as a good preparation for "the real sex" of vaginal penetration. While some former students dismissed the activity as "wasting time," Sampa was enthusiastic in his appreciation of one of his girlfriends' expertise at fellatio. He did not reciprocate. In his view, cunnilingus was something a man only did for his wife, "if at all." Dominic was alone in noting that many of those who practiced oral sex thought that this was a way of avoiding HIV, which they understood could only be transmitted through penetration of the anus or vagina

Homosexuality[17]

Oral sex, like masturbation, was also associated with homosexuality. Homosexual activity was strongly condemned by the majority of men, whether churchgoers or not—both when we spoke at the end of their schooldays and in later life. As I noted in chapter 1, same-sex attraction was commonly perceived to be a perversion of white men. To be a black or "African" man and to desire other men for most former students was a contradiction in terms. Doyal et al. (2008: 177) report the consequent tensions, because of this identification of homosexuality with white men, experienced by men in the African diaspora resident in London who desired sex with other men. At twenty, Kangwa's opinion was that homosexual activity was "even more evil than just fornicating." His views had not altered some twenty years later. Neither had Mutinta's. He repeatedly described same-sex sex as "absolutely disgusting, against nature." For some men it was a sign of insanity and they deemed homosexual men to be "inhuman."[18] The strength of feeling expressed at times acted to define hegemonic masculinity. (See Pattman [2001] for expressions of homophobia at a Zimbabwe teacher training college.)

Promise could not recall any episodes during his boyhood and adolescence of boys having sex with boys. He said he only came to learn of such activity when he was an adult. He did not consider that the boys and young men who masturbated him in his childhood were having sex with him. At his boys' primary boarding school, however, Henry was aware of same-sex activity, including anal penetration, between pupils, even though it was forbidden by an unspoken rule. While not directly involved himself, in Henry's view, it was mostly situations in which younger boys submitted to older boys and prefects in exchange for protection or privileges such as exemption from manual work. He thought perhaps 10 percent of the pupils were involved. Henry did not describe this as "homosexual," as he would later label the activity of some of his fellow students at university.

On homosexuality, the secondary religious education syllabus that students followed at St. Antony's, *Christian Living Today*, had been much less tolerant than it was about masturbation. Following a medicalized perspective, same-sex attraction was ascribed pathological origins. In discussions with me, several men were clearly anxious to distance themselves from even the remotest suspicion of a homosexual orientation. They prefaced their remarks—not unlike in discussions of witchcraft—with expressions such as "I am told." If they acknowledged knowing someone who was thought to be homosexual, they were usually at pains to stress the very tenuous nature of the acquaintance. Several former students suggested that the degree of homosexual activity in Zambia was difficult to assess because most Zambian men who engaged in homosexual activity, afraid of becoming outcasts, conducted their same-sex affairs under the cloak of a respectable heterosexual married life. Again, as when speaking of witches, men frequently observed: "These people are clever. To know them you have to be one of them." While as adolescents, they had portrayed homosexuality as a European propensity, as adults, a few former students recognized that some Zambian men might well be sexually attracted to other men. Most men offered stereotypical descriptions of homosexuals, supposedly easy to identify because of their effeminate mannerisms, their penchant for wearing earrings, and their high-pitched voices. Homosexual men were also assumed to sexually abuse boys and young men. Some men pointed to the example of a former student, known indeed for his effeminate manner while at school, who had recently completed a prison term for child abuse. Others cited an exceptionally good-looking former student who was now living in Europe.

The overwhelming majority of former students described homosexuality as "against nature," "against God," and "evil." Many men appeared genuinely puzzled by the idea that a man might be sexually attracted to another man, or even—and far more puzzling—that a woman might be attracted to another woman. Though some condemned homosexual men and lesbians outright, many declared their pity for them and expressed the hope that they might change. At twenty, Paul had dismissed homosexuality as "simply ridiculous." His conclusion that such activity was "against nature," and thus an offence against God, hardened in later life when he was Born Again. Some suggested it might be the consequence of a "strange" upbringing or drug taking. When same-sex activity was reported to take place outside the confines of prisons and boarding schools, respondents usually argued that readiness to engage in such acts was usually motivated by material gain; it was "prostitution with foreigners" for money and not the pursuit of sexual gratification. The same-sex sexual activity was normally reported to be between a younger Zambian man and an older expatriate male, often a "European." However, Lebanese men were also commonly suspected.[19]

Former students once more referenced the Bible as their "true guide." Homosexuality was in direct contravention of God's plan when he created Adam and Eve and told them to go forth and multiply. Several men made reference to the biblical Sodom and Gomorrah to illustrate God's condemnation. Suggesting a link between homosexual activity and HIV/AIDS, they commented that homosexuality was making Zambian society sick. The general opinion was that the "African gift of silence" meant that such matters were not spoken about directly and "suspects" went unchallenged. Gossip circulated and fingers were surreptitiously pointed. Examples within the family were rarely mentioned. Dominic provided an exception, describing sex between men as "very strange" when he discussed one of his uncles:

> Even from a long time ago, a long time ago, he used to sleep with boys. Well, at that time we didn't know what it meant. I mean at that time we were very young. Well, now, this time, he is successful, he has money so when he feels like having sex he says to some boy, "Okay, let's go and have sex and I will give you some money." But as for myself, I find it very strange, very strange. I don't know but there must be something very wrong with him. My uncle is married. He had two children. It was very strange. He had two girls. Okay, one passed away. The other one who is remaining is a big girl. She's about twenty. Well, I used to ask him about his behavior, "What is wrong?" He used to say, "Ah, me, well maybe a month passes and I have not had sex with my wife. I have a problem with my erection."...He has some business. He has sex with some of the boys he employs—not oral sex but anal sex.

He employs boys who look female; they look like girls. Beautiful boys are the ones he has sex with.

In contrast to most of his school contemporaries, Sampa had no particular objection to homosexuality, arguing that, while he felt no sexual interest in men, it was a legitimate sexual preference. He had never seen such things, but, like others, he thought it was a common practice among Lebanese men and that they sometimes used their wealth to seduce young Zambians. At university and during his working life Henry had had several friends who engaged in sexual activity with older, wealthier (mostly) expatriate men. One of his university contemporaries who had been sexually involved with a Greek businessman had later died. Henry was of the opinion that his friends and others who engaged in sexual activity with men were not homosexual by orientation, but rather that they got sexually involved with more powerful men for material reward. There was often an ambivalent reaction to such young Zambian men as they gained prestige because of the expensive clothes and other luxuries they acquired through such associations.[20] George had known one college student who was involved in a sexual relationship with an older white man. The European not only paid his college fees and living expenses, but also gave him a mobile phone and, in his last year of studies, provided him with the use of a car. At twenty, Simon had also been aware of some same-sex activity among his age-mates but he could not understand the attraction and objected to the practice on health grounds. Later, as a health professional, Simon noted the public silence around homosexuality in Zambia. Describing homosexual activity as "not nice sex," Simon was also of the view that most such activity was motivated by the desire for money.

Hambayi, at twenty, had judged homosexual activity to be particularly reprehensible. He knew a missionary who engaged in sexual acts—usually masturbation—with students. Hambayi expressed suspicion of any male who was unmarried or who did not seem to have sex with women, "Then just know that there is something!"[21] As for celibate Catholic missionaries, Hambayi was convinced that there were things going on in "dark corners" in this and other churches in Zambia. At forty he still condemned homosexual practice in the strongest possible terms, now blaming homosexuals for the spread of the HIV virus: "These people must be punished by God because they have gone against nature. Maybe these are the people who have brought these mysterious diseases." Homosexuality was "not in order."

God created man and woman and procreation was the main purpose. Now, why should you take your fellow sex? It's wrong!"

Simooya and Sanjoba, discussing extensive male-to-male sex in Kamfinsa Prison in Zambia where no condoms were available for prisoners, observe: "Inmates attributed male-to-male sex to sexual needs, lengthy stays at the prison, bullying and poor prison diet. Because of the erratic food supply, inmates with access to food were said to use this to obtain sexual partners" (2001: 242). A former student had served time in prison and had become aware of same-sex activity. His experience led him to conclude that it was difficult to resist the sexual demands of more powerful fellow prisoners:

> Sodomy is there; it takes a man to say no to it. Those who are loose, those who are weak, those who want to eat do that. Those who sodomize have access to goods. Those who were sodomizing others were getting food from prison officers and they used this food as bait to get fellow prisoners to have sex with them.... There were no condoms available. I never saw one. Out of every ten inmates, I would say three or four were involved in sodomy. Prison was the worst experience I have ever undergone.

Darius condemned homosexual activity, though he felt sympathy for homosexuals and hoped that they might change and become "normal." Like Sampa, he acknowledged that some men might well be attracted to other men—and women to women—arguing that their sexual activity might not be a transaction engaged in on either side simply for material gain. He knew a teenager who told him that he had been sexually abused by a German expatriate. Darius excitedly recalled his own fear when, while traveling on business, he was approached by a man for sex:

> It was, it is, a very awkward thing. In Zimbabwe a white man wanted to have sex with me. He approached me in a nightclub. At first he bought me a beer; I thought it was just a favor. Later, when I went to the toilet he followed me. He was talking like a lady and tried to start touching my penis. I screamed, ran out of the toilet, jumped in the car and drove off.

"African Infidelity"

There was almost complete agreement among men and women that "African" husbands were more unfaithful to their wives than "European" husbands were to theirs. Like others, Sampa explained

"African infidelity" by referring to the practical arrangements of everyday married life:

> I mean in Africa, it's very difficult for a man to be faithful to one wife. It's really, really difficult. Your side [Europe], I think, it's different. As for you people if you've got a wife or a girlfriend, you are always moving together—all the time. But in Africa, you must have noticed, that is very rare, very rare. The wife can be somewhere and you are also somewhere drinking. You are not together all the time so you have more opportunities.

Sampa almost never "moved with" his wife, Ruth. Most of his absences from her side in his leisure time were because he was drinking with friends, or because he was engaged in a sexual encounter elsewhere. However, he told me that I should not conclude that his relationships with other women meant that he loved his wife any the less. Again he framed his explanation in terms of supposed "racial" difference:

> You know, we Africans, it doesn't mean that if we make love to another lady—it doesn't mean that we don't love our wife. The way I understand it—I do love my wife. And even the things I do with those girlfriends—the way we have sex—it's very different from the way I perform my duties with my wife.

Promise offered very similar views. He loved his wife, and he often thought about her when they were separated. However, his love did not rule out relationships with other women:

> You know, we Africans, plenty of us Africans, well, it doesn't mean that if you make love to another lady—it doesn't mean that you really don't love your wife. I think I have that romantic idea of love, but I'll put it this way. Us Africans, or us Zambians especially, I would say, our love mostly is for sex. Personally, I love my wife. I am in love with her. It's only (laughing), it's only that I do misbehave when I am out [away from home]. (Laughing.) I accept that. (Laughing.)

Among the men interviewed, opinion was divided about whether it was more difficult for a man to control his sexual desires than for a woman. In their recent survey on the Zambian Copperbelt Muvandi et al. (n.d.) report that the general view was that it was easier for a woman. For many men it was simply a matter of biology. Men became sexually aroused much quicker than women, and therefore needed more frequent "release" and "relief." Men's much-vaunted claims of "superiority" over "weak" women were contradicted when sexual self-control was at issue. George noted, "From my experience, I am the one mostly asking for sex. My wife can go for a long time without sex—even a month. Women have a lot of self-control." Almost all men spoke about how their sexual desire was awakened by the way women dressed. Dominic described how when he saw a woman "dressed in a very funny, a very modern, way," his mind would start racing. Try as he might to resist, his desire for sex would have to be satisfied. He suggested that one reason why people were not changing their sexual behavior, in spite of the heavy toll that AIDS was taking daily in Zambia, was because "sex has got a very strong—and a very strange—drive amongst us Zambians. I personally have been a victim, a victim of this drive."

Even Peter, who had described himself to me as "somehow lame" because of his premarital sexual inexperience, spoke about how quickly he became sexually aroused by the sight of women in "European" clothes: "It's when I can see the woman's thighs, well, starting from the knees going upwards. Also the pant can be seen when the skirt is too tight. So, emotionally I imagine I am already in bed with such a person (laughing)." Darius, along with one or two other men, reported that he had discussed this matter with his wife: "I have asked her whether women get tempted or feel attracted to men on the streets like we do to women. She says they don't unless they get involved in a relationship. From that angle men and women are different. Men seem to act on impulse. We think through our manhood [penis] while women think through the mind."

Some men added notions of respectability, of gender propriety, as Malama's comments indicate:

> It's easier for a woman to control herself. I say so because a woman cannot—a respectable woman, of course, I am talking about a respectable woman—a woman cannot go out in the street to look for a man so that they sleep together. And secondly I feel that their sexual desire is not as much as us men. Where a man is concerned, yah, it's disastrous! I am saying this because I am a man and I have experienced a few things here and there. It so happens that when a man wants to have a woman, he'll make sure that he has a woman. If I am sexually starved, and I feel that on this night I must have sex, well, I will make sure that I am going to have that sex, maybe by going around taverns—trying to explore all angles until by the end of the day I'll come up with a partner. But as for women, they have reservations.

While many former students judged African men to have less control over their sexual desires than European men, some read this as a sign of superior "sexual strength." While other men saw premature ejaculation as a problem, Darius was alone in claiming this as further evidence of greater African virility: "I feel we Africans are stronger. From the blue movies I find that it takes whites too long to ejaculate because me, I would even release in less than twenty seconds. For whites it takes long. There have been moments when I have released before entering inside!"

A number of men spoke about times when their wives and other sexual partners initiated sex play and demanded sexual satisfaction. These experiences caused them to qualify their assessments about women's control of their sexual appetites. Hambayi thought the question of sexual control was "fifty-fifty." He offered to take me one night to Church Road in Lusaka to see "naked women who have failed to control themselves," offering sex for money.[22] Edmund held similar views, though, like many men and women, he spoke of the need for willpower and self-control. He was critical of some of his colleagues who, on their first night working away from home, were eager to secure the comforts of home: "You can go out [go away] for two days, but I don't think the need can arise in two days or three days, not even a week. But the first night you will go out, somebody will go to a bar and pick up a prostitute. Would you say it was out of a need? No! It is what he *wants*."

Paul also spoke of how readily his coworkers sought sex with other women when they were working for even a few days away from home. He would warn them of the dangers of AIDS and encourage them to use condoms, to which they would respond, "Don't worry, we'll use two." Some men, especially those Born Again like Paul, explicitly invoked God's help. One of the fruits of the Spirit of the living God, they told me, was self-control. When a man was without the Spirit, it was impossible for him to control his sexual desires, they said.

From his experience, Sampa had no doubt that it was more difficult for a man to control his sexual appetite. He thought women could easily live for two or three months without a sexual partner. As for himself, at forty, he "needed to have sex at least three or four times a week." Even when his wife was available, he sought additional sexual satisfaction. In times of illness, Sampa thought it was impossible for him to live without sex. He continued to have unprotected sex, even though there were indications that he was developing full-blown AIDS. Only when he was extremely ill did Sampa find that his desire for sex lessened. Starting to recover from his first bout of TB, he began to have "wet dreams." He commented to me: "Ah, no, now this is really useless. It's better that I perform on a human being.

(Laughing.) In deep sleep, you have those feelings, but they are not how it is when you do it 'live.' "[23] Sampa said that he found it very difficult to sleep without first having sexual intercourse. He very quickly resumed sexual relations with three women, one of them "organized" for him by a male friend. In Sampa's accounts, women sometimes took the lead in proposing a sexual relationship. Wives would organize meetings when their husbands were away. When they were pregnant with their husband's child, they felt freer to have unprotected sex with him.

While *in theory* Promise thought that the question of control was the same for men and women, in practice he had found that it had been impossible for him to forego extramarital relationships. The urgency of his desire overrode any lingering suspicion that there might be some truth in the "traditional" teaching he had received before marriage that the health of a child in the womb or an infant at the breast might be put at risk by the father's infidelity. Promise explained that, despite intentions to abstain from extramarital sex, he was "easily tempted" by the sight of a woman. He also recognized the influence of his best friend, Mwanza. His friend would encourage him to have sex with as many different women as he himself did, and, Promise maintained, would stimulate his own desire by open displays of affection toward women they met in bars: "If you happen to see your friend with a lady and they are kissing each other, well, just by seeing what is going on, you are also stimulated. You think also of having a lady. You are forced!"

Promise recognized his fears about appearing weak:

> When there is no lady around, I don't even think of it. But there are times when I reverse my emotions when I am with a lady.... I don't know whether I have that feeling, Well, if I don't do it, then the lady might think I am weak—that I have become weak—that I cannot go out with [have sex with] her. I mean my manhood—it's about strength, strength.

During 2002 Promise's friend, Mwanza, died of AIDS. The three of us had met together quite often. Promise concluded that Mwanza had "lost hope of his life." Mwanza's first wife had left him. She had had several extramarital relationships, including one with the local bank manager and was now engaged in a number of sexual liaisons with local men. She was believed to be the source of the local gossip that Mwanza was "not a man," that he was impotent. Promise thought that Mwanza's second marriage was his attempt to scotch the rumors. Mwanza had also had several other sexual partners during his first marriage. Mwanza's second wife had been seriously ill even before they married. She became very thin and developed large blisters (Kaposi's sarcoma) over her body. She died in 2001. She had been diagnosed with TB; Mwanza was convinced that her death was AIDS-related. Haunted by the thought that he might well be HIV-positive, Mwanza became more and more despondent. Drinking heavily, he had a number of sexual encounters. Promise commented, "Now, he has that feeling that he has AIDS as well—so he does not [take] care of his life and he is a man who is irresponsible." Promise tried to advise his friend. In my company, Mwanza always conducted himself in a very deferential manner when he was sober and did his best to hide from me when he was drunk. When sober, Mwanza appeared to listen to Promise's warnings of the risks he was taking, but when he was drunk, he angrily rejected what he perceived to be interference in his life. One evening he had a woman in the room he was occupying in Lusaka. He had picked her up at a bar. The woman had demanded that he use condoms. On his "second round" the condom burst. He told me that he had "released inside" the woman. It was only when he asked the woman to clean his penis, she realized that the condom had burst. A fierce argument ensued, the woman accusing him; "You have already killed me now. What are you doing?" Fueled by alcohol, the argument raged for some time, but they were eventually reconciled. They later decided to take a shower together and in the shower they had intercourse once more, this time without a condom. Mwanza commented afterward, "Us, we are already dead! Using condoms now, it's useless. Yes, *twali fwa kalee.* [We died some time ago]."

Alcohol contributed to men's low levels of male condom use in extramarital sex. (See also Ndubani 2002: 37.) All men claimed that beer stimulated their sexual appetite. Many automatically associated drinking in bars with having casual sex. Beer gave men such as Promise and Sampa "courage" to approach women for sex. They recognized that beer released their inhibitions. Promise told me that once the effects of the beer wore off, the "courage" evaporated, to be replaced, at least temporarily, by anxiety about the possibility of contracting the HIV virus. Some men explained that they reduced the risk of unprotected casual sex by having sexual intercourse with their wives *before* they went to drink beer. They might still be "tempted" but they were already sexually satisfied, they explained. In this way they felt protected.

Conclusion

Africa has a long history of the constructions of "difference" based upon supposedly discrete sexualities and moralities. In her analysis of responses to syphilis in colonial East and Central Africa, Vaughan documents how assumptions of moral disintegration and dangerous female sexuality led the British at first to ignore evidence that the disease was present in an endemic, non-venereally transmitted form. She comments: "We have only to turn to the 1980s, and to representations of the African AIDS epidemic, to recognize that social constructions of disease remain (and will always remain) powerful, and that a century of colonial rule and of a medicalized discourse on the 'African' has had lasting effects" (1992: 299). Pigg and Adams note the ways in which "gendered sexuality has functioned as a symbolic site for the elaboration of group boundaries and differences and it continues to function as such under postcolonial nationalisms" (2005: 9). In their critique of programs that objectify sex and sexuality "in the name of well-being," they observe that we should not expect to find any simple confrontation between modern and indigenous values. Graduates of St. Antony's used sexuality as a marker to draw a boundary between "Europeans" and "Africans," white and black, modernity and tradition, men and women, adults and children. However, such boundaries often became blurred when they strategically raided "tradition" to justify their power and their demands for sexual satisfaction. Most men identified an "African sexuality"—a notion that some mobilized self-critically as an instance of "African backwardness," but that others claimed as the moral high ground against immoral Europeans who flaunted their sexuality and engaged in unacceptable practices such as homosexuality.

Men did not necessarily accept the constructions of "sex" that HIV/AIDS campaigns promoted. "Sex," "the real thing," was nothing less than penetrative vaginal intercourse. It was this that gave men a feeling of achievement. For the majority, condoms denied them a sense of completion; they felt they had not really "met" their partner. Ideally, intercourse should entail "skin-to-skin" contact. In addition to some women's complaints about wasting semen, men said that women needed to feel the semen entering their bodies. Numerous men spoke of their uneasiness when they ejaculated into a condom—and not only because of the loss of sensation. For them, semen became matter-out-of place, if it was not deposited inside a woman. Some men feared that their semen might be used in love potions to lure them away from their wives, or even in witchcraft attacks against them. The threat of AIDS appeared, at least temporarily, to recede.

Men's sexual experience transformed with the passage of time and the consequent physical changes in their bodies. In contrast to their youthful accounts, many more spoke of their need to satisfy their partners sexually. Some had come to enjoy "taking time in sex." This was not simply in order to "keep" the women for themselves, but because "fairness should prevail": women had the right to expect their partner to attend to their needs and desires. Adult masculinity was intimately expressed in this way. However, the shadow cast by AIDS led few men to be sufficiently sensitive to women's vulnerability as to seek to protect them from possible HIV transmission, by, for example, using condoms during intercourse.

Men's pleasure certainly figured heavily in their rejection of condoms as it had in their youth. Very few men had any experience of the female condom; there was little enthusiasm for it either among men or women. Several wives had been given female condoms at government clinics, but few couples had actually tried them, and none were using them on a regular basis. Women feared that a female condom might get stuck inside their bodies. They also objected to their color and wondered why they could not be made to match their skin tone. The few men who had tried them complained that they were "noisy" and their fear of loss of control over their semen seemed heightened. Performance anxieties remained, as "sexual strength" had to be demonstrated. Some men continued to worry that using condoms prevented speedy "rounds." Many men were well aware that men's claim of conquest was little more than a pretence. They knew that it was not always men who went after women; women might well go after men. Men's all-conquering assertions masked for many a fear of appearing weak. The powerful gaze of their peer group was never far away.

Women might do as they had been taught by *banacimbusa* and endeavor to make themselves dry out of "respect" for men, and to ensure men's comfort and pleasure, though this did not imply that they would not seek sexual satisfaction for themselves. They might also, once more, become men's tutors in such "modern" sexual techniques as oral sex. Money brought some former students "excitement" and what they saw as greater opportunities for extramarital affairs. Because of HIV/AIDS, some former students told me, a man had to be "courageous" when "hunting for women." Beer gave men "courage" to approach women for sex. For most men, adult sexual desire continued to be felt as an urgent need that had to be repeatedly satisfied. With their hydraulic model of African male sexuality, they spoke of their need to seek "release," to feel "relief." They at times felt "driven" to find "sex," whatever the risks. They portrayed this as an absence of control, while still claiming their right, as men, to be in command in sexual relations. This is not to deny that they also considered some sexual intercourse as a deep expression of love. Though many enjoyed affectionate relationships with their wives and other women, men became strikingly inarticulate when I asked them to describe what "love," the love of wives and girlfriends, meant for them. With regard to their marriage, they cited as expressions of love the care they received from their wives and the efforts they, in turn, made to provide materially for their families. While former students experienced a range of feelings in their relationships with women, they seemed to have a restricted vocabulary of emotions, at least in English, to convey them. Their need to be "understood" in these relationships was clearly uppermost for many men, as it had been in their youth. As for their embodied sexual experience, many told me that intercourse was the most enjoyable experience a human being could have, but beyond that they were silent. Many cautioned me against concluding that their extramarital affairs meant that they did not love their wives. They countered my initial attempts to discuss the risks of HIV infection they created for their wives by their unprotected extramarital sexual intercourse with such comments as "This has got nothing to do with my wife" and "Why are you bringing my wife into this?" However, while many came to acknowledge these risks, few saw any easy solution. Marriage became a problem in this regard. Some men had concluded, without having an HIV test, that they were already HIV-positive. Using a condom would "make no difference now," they intimated.

God told Adam, "Go forth and multiply," former students reminded me—as they had done twenty years previously. They saw no contradiction between God's injunction in Genesis and their wives' use of contraception. Perhaps this was because the pill and injectable contraception that their partners took (and which men judged made their use of condoms unnecessary) did not interfere with their masculine performance of "sex," that is, penetrative intercourse with their semen deposited in its "proper" place, inside their partner.[24] Men judged *some* sexual acts that did not leave open the possibility of procreation to be immoral. Adult solitary masturbation, for example, fell into this category, though men also saw this as an expression of "selfishness."[25] Mutual masturbation might be enjoyed as a "warm up" to "sex," the "real thing," but it was no substitute, and could not be countenanced as a strategy of HIV risk reduction.

The Bible provided former students with a rich rhetorical resource through which to judge the morality of particular sex acts. Strongest condemnation was reserved for homosexuality—evidenced by widespread homophobia and by some men's readiness to make homosexual men the scapegoats for the AIDS pandemic in Africa. Such homophobia has been widely reported in sub-Saharan Africa. Morrell and Swart (2005: 97) have noted how it has become a feature of African nationalism as articulated by such leaders as Robert Mugabe in Zimbabwe and Sam Nujoma in Namibia. For former students, moral acts were "natural" acts. God created the world and all that was in it—indeed God and "nature" at times appeared to be almost synonymous. I next turn to explore former students' religious ideas.

7

"Has God Come in Another Way?"

No consideration of contemporary life in Zambia can afford to omit the role of religion. Yet, what constitutes religious belief and religious identity? What is the relationship, if any, between religious belief and church membership and between these and the way a person acts in the world? What are the consequences of these for decision-making in sexual activity, for AIDS prevention, stigma reduction, care of the sick and the dying? This chapter explores the attempts of former students and their wives to make sense of the AIDS pandemic.

The cost of AIDS in Zambia in terms of loss and grief, as well as in material terms, has been devastating. Former students' mothers, wives, and sisters, who did most of the physical caring for AIDS sufferers in their homes, repeatedly spoke of the shame of dying from AIDS. In part, this was because of the assumed association between AIDS and "promiscuity." When Kabwe was dying with all the signs of what appeared to be AIDS, he was at pains to insist to me and his family and friends, "It's not AIDS." Having multiple sexual partners was judged as evidence of "immorality" and "sinfulness" and promiscuity implied greater risk of infection.[1] There appeared to be little recognition that a person might have multiple partners but reduce the risk through using condoms, or that intercourse with a single partner might well entail the risk of contracting HIV. AIDS deaths were considered to be particularly shameful because of the attendant physical deterioration and the loss of control of bodily functions. Incontinence in adults, which rendered them the status of infants, was singled out as the most distressing and degrading aspect of such "undignified" deaths. Elizabeth, Chimbala's widow, spoke movingly about her husband's AIDS-related death, two years earlier, and of how it had provided an avenue of escape from an abusive relationship. At first Chimbala had refused to discuss the possibility that his progressively serious illnesses might be AIDS-related. Following his death, Elizabeth, like many Zambians, employed expressions such as "I think" and the subjunctive voice as she gently conveyed her conviction—correct as events subsequently revealed—that she was HIV-positive. A university graduate in her early thirties, working for a local council, Elizabeth described how she learned about her husband's illness:

> I became aware of his status when one doctor told me that my husband's problem was also mine. My mind opened. I got tired of looking after him. I think it was AIDS that killed my husband. First he had diarrhea, then fevers in the night. He was put on TB treatment, but then it was terminated. Then he had meningitis. He had a lumbar puncture but he died before the results came out. He used to boast that he had had an HIV test and it was negative and he said that if he became positive, I would be the one responsible. The death of my husband was a relief because my life with him was not happy. When he was dying, I had packed my things. He had become so abusive and his mother would join in. But he was the kind of person who would abuse you but would never let go.... He used to beat me. I have the scars. Once I got my gratuity.[2] We made a budget together. I was paying for his course from the U.K. When we went to cash the check we found that the pound had become too powerful. Anyway, I gave him the money to pay *Supreme Furnishers* [a popular furniture store where items could be bought on credit] and so on. He came back drunk and started beating me. I had just lost my father. I nearly cut his throat. I packed my things and took my son to my brother's place.... After my husband's death, my things were almost grabbed by his relatives. I had to get the help of the police. I have lost two houses. This experience has given me strength.

Mutinta was one of many former students who spoke of the depression that at times overwhelmed him:

> I've had to get used to it. It affects me in the sense that it makes me realize how short life is. It is a terrible thing that now people die much earlier than they used to. And this AIDS is affecting rich and poor alike. It is so depressing that I would rather not concentrate on it. I have seen too many depressing cases. If I thought about them too much I would get sick.

Mutinta's wife, Mutale, spoke in a similar way: "I really don't know who is an AIDS patient and who isn't, but we have lost relatives and friends. I feel pity. I feel bad when I see people misbehaving when there is so much suffering. It has affected me. I have seen so many relatives and close friends suffer."

Henry's wife, Pamela, spoke of the pain she experienced watching the suffering that AIDS brought: "I and my husband have lost close family members. My brother-in-law was in and out of hospital and I saw him shrink. I knew that it was HIV, and one of his sisters confirmed it. The pain he went through was really touching; to see someone you joked and laughed with waste away and die!"

Sampa described the difficulty relatives had in accepting that someone was suffering from AIDS-related conditions because of stigma and the sense of hopelessness that accompanied the pandemic. He gave the example of a cousin's husband. In trying to help, he got drawn into family quarrels:

> It was confirmed, it was TB-AIDS. Now this other day me and my brother-in-marriage we decided to take him to the hospital. So they told us, "This man is suffering from this and this." So when we came back I told my in-law [mother-in-law] and everybody. So there was a quarrel. "Ah, you! How can you tell someone is suffering from TB? Are you a doctor? Ah, these things you have told us!" They started insulting us. Even the man himself said, "You, ah, how can you be telling me that I am suffering from TB? You are not a doctor!" And then his wife, my cousin, started insulting me. They had told him in the hospital that it was TB. He even lied to them at home, but I told them, "This is the situation." Now the wife also got upset. So I said, "Look there's nothing to do." He was a door-bouncer. So that's where—it even explained the AIDS, you know, such jobs, you are always meeting ladies there.

The man died in hospital and Sampa had first to get the burial permit and then go to the hospital to collect the corpse. He had to enter the mortuary and search for the body. Judging that he risked infection, Sampa bought a pair of plastic gloves at the mortuary. Accusations and recriminations followed the burial. The family of the deceased man accused the widow of having killed her husband. They said that she had given him AIDS because she was "too movious" (she had multiple partners). She retaliated by accusing her dead husband of bringing AIDS into their home. It was common knowledge in the neighborhood that he regularly returned from the nightclub with different women, while his wife was out at work.

Religious Ideas

The teenage religious ideas of the original cohort of former students about God and the problem of evil and suffering have significance for adult understandings of HIV/AIDS. All the men in this study identified themselves as Christians, most of them third generation. However, this did not necessarily mean they accepted much of the Christian teaching they were offered. While most imagined some form of afterlife, few students accepted the existence of heaven, hell, purgatory, or the resurrection of Jesus, and even fewer, the doctrine of the Virgin Birth, a particularly puzzling teaching. Like most students, Paul had thought that hell was merely "an invention of Christians to frighten people." Baptized a Catholic in infancy, he was convinced in his teens that he would die young and he told me that there had to be, however, some kind of afterlife. Most self-identified Catholics did not accept the transubstantiation of the bread and wine into the body and blood of Christ at Mass, but took Communion. Few former students remained regular churchgoers once they left St. Antony's, once they had escaped the surveillance of church-going parents, though they expected their children to attend church.

At school, all the students I interviewed asserted some belief in God or a Supreme Being, though for the majority Jesus was a shadowy figure. Most described God as a personal deity. Concepts of God are open to change, as people puzzle over the meaning of human life in the light of their own experience. Colson (2004) and Hinfelaar (1994) have explored the history of Tonga and Bemba notions of God (*Leza/Lesa*). In many respects these commentators portray a similar picture. They both suggest that dramatic shifts occurred with the entry of Christian missionaries into the region, though their arrival was just one element in rapidly changing societies. Only *Leza*, of all the spiritual forces that Tonga recognized, was acceptable to become absorbed and thereby to convey missionary ideas about their Christian God. Colson reports that in the 1940s her Tonga informants stressed the human inability adequately to conceptualize *Leza* who had no material form, neither shrines, nor priests. They told her: "'*Leza* is like the wind. We do not see wind. We do not know what wind is. We feel wind on our bodies. We see trees bend. We know it by what it does'" (2004: 2). *Leza* was not normally thought responsible for illness and death. Indeed, *Leza* remained the very last resort when all other explanations failed. "People said, '*Leza*, what else?' or '*Leza* laughed.'" *Leza*'s primary role was that of creator and as such *Leza* was assumed to be beneficent and benevolent. Creation was not seen to lead to a further end. Hinfelaar describes a range of Bemba deities, among them *Mulenga wa Mpanga* and *Ngulu*. Many were originally associated with the natural world and with a creator of the world who once dwelt among humans. Various myths explained the creator's withdrawal from the world, often placing the blame squarely upon women. Bantu languages do not use gender as a grammatical category; the Tonga Creator *Leza* had no gender (Colson 2004: 2), while the Bemba *Lesa* possessed both the male and female mode of being human, often invoked as *Mayo na Tata* (mother and father) (Hinfelaar 1994: 6). However, for St. Antony's students there was no doubt about the gender of God: God was masculine. The created world, the earth, the sun, the moon, and human beings remained convincing testimonies of the existence and the power of God. For young men, only a masculine God could have such power. As a teenager, Darius commented to me, "When I was young, I used to think that God looked something like my father." Given the difficult relationships that many former students had with their fathers in childhood and adolescence, a readiness on the part of some to accept the idea of a God who punished, rather than one who comforted, is perhaps unsurprising.

At school, as in later life, almost all preferred the biblical account of creation to the Darwinian theory of evolution. The young men regularly cited the Book of Genesis where God creates Adam *first* as evidence of male superiority, explaining that in this instance Christianity and "tradition" were as one. Maleness was automatically deserving of respect. As in so much of everyday Zambian life, precedence was all-important and there was no doubt that Eve, the woman, came second.[3] Few students expressed belief in the existence of the soul portrayed in Christian dogma, though many used the term "sin" when speaking of their sexual activity. With some exceptions, this seemed simply to imply wrongful action that carried no particular consequences. For example, Catholic students did not feel any need to confess this sin, or any other sin to a priest. With the exception of those who belonged to Pentecostal denominations, the majority of students felt that what they considered their normal premarital sexual activity was no concern of the church.

Most students assured me that God intervened in human life. At school, many related how they had experienced God's help in passing exams.[4] They had prayed to him and he had answered them. For some, the very fact that they had managed to get a mission education and to gain academic qualifications even though they had come from poor backgrounds, struggling to get sufficient financial support for school requisites, transport money, and examination fees, was proof enough of God's care. As a teenager, Kangwa prayed to God in moments of crisis such as when his girlfriend's period was late. In childhood, he had suffered poor health. He was at first persuaded by his mother's suspicions that her own mother was the cause of his chest problems. At the end of his schooldays he explained to me that, as he had grown older, he had become increasingly skeptical. He had rejected his mother's diagnosis and concluded that his ill-health, like his poverty, was God's punishment because he had not been "very dedicated" to God: he had engaged in premarital sex. However, Kangwa considered that God was unfair in punishing *him* when others, in his view "equally unfaithful," enjoyed good health and prosperity. Though Kangwa would stop attending church after school, he would continue to identify himself as a Catholic. At forty and in ill-health, not a churchgoer, he still asserted that God existed. In his youth he had consoled himself with the thought that the "unfaithful" who had enjoyed this life would meet their punishment in the next. In adulthood, such solace was no longer available to him, now that he had rejected the idea of an afterlife.

Christian missionaries introduced the figure of Satan into the region in the late nineteenth century.[5] In adolescence, many students rejected the idea of Satan. If Satan *did* exist and caused men to commit evil, other students reasoned, then Satan was God's responsibility. At school, Kangwa was not the only one to comment, "Sometimes God behaves strangely," an observation he would repeat some twenty years later. The conundrum for Kangwa was that God had created the world and human beings as they were and so God was responsible for evil in the world. If the Devil existed, then this was God's doing, he observed: "We cannot blame the Devil. It's absurd." When we spoke in 1984, Sampa explained that he believed in God's existence because of the natural world and the human beings in it. Baptized a Catholic in infancy, as a teenager, Sampa went to Mass regularly and he also received Communion. He rejected any idea that God might punish people in this life, though he thought God might well punish people in the world to come. People would go either to heaven or hell. Sampa expressed the majority student view when he suggested to me that Satan was simply an idea brought by Christian missionaries "to keep men and women in order."

Two students rejected the idea of a personal God who intervened in human affairs. As teenagers, Henry and his close school friend, Simon, were attracted to the idea of reincarnation. They held the view that God had programed human beings; every life-course was predetermined. (They would repeat this conviction twenty years later, while rejecting reincarnation.) Henry was raised by devout Catholic parents. Yet he rejected their conviction that God would one day judge the living and the dead, as he did any ideas of heaven and hell.

In his teens, Henry was troubled by what he described to me as "the confused picture" he found in the Bible. In our conversations just before he began his university studies, Henry expressed puzzlement as to why God should fool Adam and Eve in the Garden of Eden by asking where they were, when he knew full well. From his reading of the Bible, Henry was troubled to learn that God had even encouraged slavery. Simon offered a similar interpretation, commenting, "I don't think I need to believe in all these things."

Mutinta, brought up by devout Baptist parents, claimed there had to be a God, "a power, a greater force," because without God life would have no purpose. As a young man, Mutinta said he believed that there was heaven and hell and that those who did not believe in God would go to hell. In his youth he had anticipated that the older he grew, the more inclined he would become to believe in a "spiritual world." However, at forty he would reject the possibility of any kind of afterlife. He dismissed ideas of heaven and hell and puzzled over the problem of evil, questioning in particular the existence of the Devil: "Why did God create Lucifer, when he knew that there would be a heaven and hell? If there was some kind of judgment, who would be judged?"

At school, Hambayi described himself as someone who had never been a "strong believer" in Christian teaching. His view was that God neither helped nor punished in this life. Though he affirmed a belief in God the creator, he rejected the Genesis account of creation. (In later life Hambayi would draw on this account, especially the creation of Adam and Eve, to assert a husband's superiority over his wife and his repugnance of homosexuality.) Forced as a child and a teenager to attend the Seventh Day Adventist (SDA) Church by his father, Hambayi as a young adult had come to the conclusion that to believe in some kind of life after death was "just a psychological defeat." He stopped going to church services in his late teens. At school he had become a heavy smoker and attended beer parties,[6] able to roam out-of-bounds practically at will once he was made a school prefect. At home, his father, a polygamist, brooked no questioning of the tenets of his SDA church. Hambayi had had to remain silent about his rejection of Seventh Day Adventist teaching especially with regard to alcohol and tobacco, for fear of his father's violent reaction. He recalled, "My father would hit you with the nearest thing he could find—a piece of wood from the fire—anything!" As a teenager, Hambayi rejected any idea of personal responsibility, arguing that if there was a God, then God had made each one of us the way we were. God neither helped nor punished in this life and there was no afterlife.

However, in his early forties, Hambayi would revise some of his views in the light of painful experience. He would remain unsure about an afterlife, but he had lost his first wife, two children, his mother and father; two brothers and many close friends had died from AIDS. He would dearly love to see them again. Hambayi suspected that his suffering might be part of God's plan. He had prayed and received some guidance, though he was unsure whether this had come from God or from his late father. Still not a churchgoer, he had come to think that he should indeed find a church. He read Zambia's economic problems and the spread of AIDS as signs of the times. Death or the end of the world would surely come soon. But the problem was as follows: Which church should he join?

WITCHCRAFT

At school, some young men were convinced of the efficacy of witchcraft and the power of charms. Hambayi and Sampa suspected their fathers were witches. Darius was convinced that his uncle practiced witchcraft. Others preferred to keep an open mind, remarking that they had become "more scientific" in their thinking because of the education they received at St. Antony's. Fears of being bewitched regularly emerged in the accounts of teenage nightmares. The threat of witchcraft came from older people, sometimes the very old, who, it was assumed, would be particularly envious of the young and the abundance of life that lay ahead of them.[7] (See Auslander 1993.) Hambayi's was just one of the many nightmares I recorded:

> Here at school, preparing to go home, I had this nightmare—which I have had before. It so happened that I was dreaming that I had gone home and then there I spent a night. During the night somebody came into my hut. He came just there near my bed. He entered through the window, very fast, in a very fast move! The window is just next to where my head is when I sleep. Anyway, he hammered me here [pointing to the back of his head] on the head and then he came behind the bed. Now, that night I hadn't covered myself because I had a mosquito net. So he came behind me. I tried to scream but *zat* [nothing]. I couldn't manage. Then he came back. He tried to remove the mosquito net so that he could touch me. He had something in his hand. I don't know what it was, but I think it was medicine. I think he was trying to harm me in some way. I tried to scream. *Zat!* Nothing! At last I threw a blow but I knocked over the candle and the candlestick holder that I had put on a chair by the side of my bed. Everything fell. I woke up.

Paul told me he was very skeptical about the existence of witches, at least, as he put it, when he was in his "right mind." In his last year at St. Antony's, he described a recurrent dream, though he sought a psychological explanation:

> The dream concerns an old couple who are neighbors. They pass our house. Somehow I fear that they are trying to bewitch me. In my dream I am walking home from hospital and I meet the old woman. She is angry and so she wants to bewitch me. Then I am at the market; the woman approaches me and then she disappears. Then my girlfriend appears and then she leaves abruptly, saying, "I am going back home. I'll come later." I have had this dream twice recently. When I wake up, I don't feel okay. To me the dream is inexplicable. Perhaps it's my feeling of insecurity.

Many students had received "traditional medicine," especially in infancy and childhood; they bore its marks in the form of scars on their bodies from small razor cuts. Some of this medicine, they understood, had been given to them as protection against witchcraft attacks. Rural childhoods, in particular, had afforded opportunities to witness the activities of witch-finders and to hear the confessions of, usually elderly, villagers identified as witches. At the heart of understandings of the activity of witches was the general agreement that it was the nature of a human being to be "jealous," that is envious. Students identified the African capacity for "jealousy" as the cause of most suffering. The greatest threat came from within the extended family. Witchcraft demonstrated the dark side of kinship (Geschiere and Fisiy 1994: 325). Students claimed that "Africans" had a tendency to be more envious of fellow "Africans" than of "Europeans." It was thought impossible that a European (always implicitly figured as male), with all his material advantages and economic power, would ever be envious of a black man. The common student view was, "Blacks are most vicious to blacks."[8] Because of this capacity for envy, fellow Zambians, especially family members, were often described as unpredictable and hence unreliable. Mothers were the only consistent exception to this rule. A common feature of life within extended families was the sharp disparities in wealth and educational opportunities. Among kin, these differences caused some to feel vulnerable to witchcraft attacks. Demba was the son of a wealthy businessman. In his teens, he described the precautions the family took before making trips back to his father's home village:

> Before we go we take some traditional medicine. My uncle [father's older brother] comes to town first and brings the medicine for us. We

all drink it. It protects us from people in the village who practice witchcraft. I don't know what the medicine is. I just see it and drink it. It's better not to take chances. Some people practice witchcraft and, you know, if you have been more successful than them in life, they don't like it. They'd like to get rid of you. It's jealousy.

As a teenager, David feared that the birth of his first child would arouse envy and anger:

> When people have their first children, other relatives are so jealous about such achievements. You know, traditionally in our society, having children is some sort of achievement and so, you know, it raises a lot of dust. A lot of people think that you have started a good life by having that child so they will try and bring you down and at least if you have your child killed when it is three or four, well, you'll feel really bad. They prefer not to have blood because they like to make it appear mysterious. They want to make it look like the person died normally—a natural death. But it is through such "natural" deaths that people have come to learn how *ndoshi* [witches] operate. People now know that these deaths are caused by witches. They find out by going to a *nganga* [witchdoctor] who tells them why the person died.

THE MEANING OF AIDS

Former students, like other Zambians, tried to comprehend the HIV/AIDS crisis within the terms of their prior experience and understandings of illness, suffering, and misfortune. Men and women struggled to cope with the consequences of the pandemic on a day-to-day basis. What were the origins of the pandemic? Could they find any meaning in HIV/AIDS? What was God's role, if any, in this scene of human suffering? There was no consensus; for many no single explanation sufficed. The men and women in this study rejected the Christian notion of the redemptive value of human suffering. Some said diseases just happened and that HIV/AIDS was a disease like any other. Others maintained that diseases were "sent for human beings." Who could know for certain? Uncertainty at times may well be preferable to knowing. Reynolds-Whyte (1997) sensitively explores the consequences for explanations of HIV/AIDS in eastern Uganda, highlighting the pragmatics of uncertainty. She argues that a biomedical HIV-positive diagnosis leaves no room for negotiation; unlike the actions of spirits and witches, there is no agent of misfortune that can be addressed. Rather than learn what is assumed to be a death sentence, patients and relatives prefer the subjunctive voice that denotes other possibilities or the unknown. This opting for "uncertainty" was evident both in relation to deaths caused by AIDS and in former students' resistance to campaigns encouraging people to know their HIV status.

A few former students, though none of their wives, suspected that HIV/AIDS was part of a white (American) conspiracy to kill blacks, a suspicion reported widely throughout the region.[9] Some men suggested that the statistics produced by UNAIDS and other Western agencies were grossly inflated in order to pathologize Africa (considered a time-honored European propensity) and to justify what many increasingly saw as an AIDS industry. Others were convinced that the situation was worsening and that Zambians were "living in a coffin." Economic decline and the ravages of AIDS were read as mirror images of the health, or rather sickness, of the country and many recognized how economics and health were inextricably intertwined.

Historians have observed that epidemics have provoked similar responses in very different historical and geographical contexts, though the relationship between epidemics and ideas about them is complex (Slack 1992: 3). However, exploring responses to past famines in East Africa and the present crisis of AIDS, Lonsdale (2007: 146) notes striking contrasts both in the profiles of victims and in resulting stigmatization. He suggests that while survival strategies in the past tended to be based around the individual or the household it is possible to discern the beginnings of strategies, if not of survival, at least of prolonging life, that are assertive and more collective. In his discussion of innovative prophetic responses to epidemics in eastern and southern Africa during the late nineteenth- and early twentieth century, Ranger (1992) identifies three ideological responses—the biomedical, the so-called "traditional" African religion, and Islam and Christianity. He stresses the importance of recognizing not only the tensions *between* them but also *within* each of them (ibid.: 242). Charting colonial medical ideas on venereal diseases in East and Central Africa, Vaughan (1992: 301) notes the importance, and the difficulty, of trying to discern changing representations and responses to these diseases in African communities, and in particular, the influence of Christianity on constructions of sexuality. Jeater has argued, "Perhaps the biggest charge that can be leveled against the colonial occupiers of Southern Rhodesia is that of the serpent in the Garden of Eden: they brought the concept of 'sin,' of individual sexual shame, into societies which had not used the idea before" (1993: 266). As I have indicated, in their youth only some former students appeared to accept the concept of "sin" in terms of individual sexual shame. Perhaps this is because it has been easier for men, unlike women, to escape censure in sexual matters.[10]

Few studies have attempted to examine the intersection between religion and AIDS in Africa and, in particular, to establish whether religion or religious involvement has any salience for the prevention of HIV transmission.[11] The little that has been done often employs unexamined, generalized, or nebulous terms as some researchers readily recognize. Using the concepts of "indoctrination," "religious experience," "exclusion," and "socialization," Garner (2000) reports his research in a KwaZulu township. He argues that though a large majority of South Africans are affiliated to Christian churches, only Pentecostal churches significantly reduce extra- and premarital sex among members and thus behavior likely to promote HIV transmission.[12] Discourses that reject the biomedical explanations for the transmission of HIV, and the teachings of some religious groups, have commonly been judged by "development" agencies to be a major hindrance to the successful delivery of prevention campaigns. Other people's "culture" has been perceived as a major obstacle (Frankenberg 1995). Exploring incidents of witchfinding in southern Zambia in the mid-1990s, Bawa Yamba (1997) argues that the conjunction of biomedical, missionary and traditional discourses has caused confusion and led to a resurgence of witchcraft accusations and witchfinding activities. (See also Thomas 2007.)

AIDS OR WITCHCRAFT?

Following the burial of the husband of Sampa's cousin, some of the deceased's relatives returned to visit his grave but pointedly left immediately afterward without visiting the widow. Sampa, drawing freely on two discourses of suffering and death, became concerned about his cousin's future well-being, explaining: "You know, there's actually witchcraft when such things happen. So I was telling my sister-in-law [his cousin, the widow] 'Ah, so you are also going to die.' You see, both because of AIDS and because of witchcraft—the combination, ah, it's a deadly combination."

Some men believed that witches were artful enough to kill their victims and yet make it appear as if the cause of death was AIDS. However, this remained only one possible explanation when family and friends died. Promise had grown up in a rural area and had been aware of the activities of witches as a child. The many deaths of friends and neighbors depressed him, making him feel more vulnerable, but they did not cause him to discontinue his extramarital affairs in which he often had unprotected sex. He described his mother's fears that he was vulnerable to witchcraft attacks:

> People at home were saying those who are playing magic are the ones who wouldn't like to see people educated. You see, all those friends who died were the only ones in their families who were so educated and they all died. But, you know, those who have died, they just come home with AIDS. They come home to die. But as for me meanwhile, well I have seen those who just sit at home—they are not educated and they are also dying. So at times I am worried. When I am leaving home, my mother tells me not to say bye to anybody, "Just leave," she says, "these people are very crafty!" She means that if these people know your movements, they may find means of eliminating you by magic.

Promise heeded his mother's advice, varying the route he took on departure, always slipping away unnoticed. Like a number of other former students, at times, he suspected that *some* witchcraft attacks were made to look like AIDS. However, of the six primary school contemporaries whose recent deaths he was aware of, he attributed four of them to AIDS, one to "mental confusion," and only one to witchcraft that was made to look like AIDS.

During 2002, Promise's brother Esau became gravely ill. When Esau grew thin and was diagnosed with TB and malaria, Promise was convinced that the underlying problem was AIDS, though there remained a slight suspicion that witchcraft might be involved. As Esau's health deteriorated, Promise explained to me, "I have it in mind that it is AIDS, though I am not sure. Others suspect witchcraft." Esau's parents, like many neighbors, concluded that Esau was dying from AIDS, as did Esau himself. While Esau's mother kept her diagnosis within the immediate family, Esau's father, with whom Esau had recently quarreled, told all and sundry. At the local rural health center, there was no explicit discussion with Esau about the possibility of AIDS, even though the first of his three wives had died from what had been assumed to be AIDS, and his second wife was unwell. As his condition deteriorated and he grew thinner and thinner, Esau told Promise that he thought he was suffering from AIDS. Esau had seen several family members and neighbors die in a similar way. Promise secretly agreed with his brother's diagnosis, though he did not tell him. He suspected that the refusal of the medical officer to name his brother's disease was motivated by compassion. "They don't say it's AIDS because they think maybe that person will lose hope, will die earlier. So he was not told." Promise did his best to encourage Esau and to offer him hope:

> I am trying to discourage him from the idea, "No, it's not AIDS. Any time you will get healed." That is what I am telling him. "No, I am dying, I am dying!" "No, you won't die. You'll get healed. You just keep taking that medicine. You will be ok." But, ah, (laughing), ah, in a way I know it is AIDS.

After quarrelling with his third wife, Esau was taken to his mother's home. On extended visits to his mother's home, Promise took his share of caring for his brother, sleeping beside him at night. Afraid that he might contract his brother's illness, his mother bought some rubber gloves for Promise to wear when touching and holding his brother. After Esau's death, Promise retained the conviction that AIDS had killed his brother, though within the family rumors of witchcraft, based largely on what Promise's sister revealed in possession trances, remained. Promise explained:

> My sister was trying to reveal some things to us, to my mother, that is. I wasn't there. Now, this other sister of mine who was there, she says, "No, the brother was sick quite alright, but it had not reached when he was supposed to die." You see, the elder sister to the [my] mum, she's a witch, according to her explanation. Now this auntie of mine had bewitched somebody some time back, had killed somebody some time back. Now these others were saying that they wanted to revenge on one of her relations. Now this aunt decided that they kill the [my] brother. Now, when they killed the brother, these others were complaining that my brother's meat was bitter because he was already finished [wasted away] so they want to kill another one from our family. Now, my sister, when she came to visit me, she told me, "Mum said, don't ever pass by her place. They will clear you! They will kill you!" I will be bewitched. But I was telling them, "No. There is no way they can bewitch me. Why?" "No, the meat of that one that they killed, it was bitter, so we never enjoyed that meat. So we are still looking for someone to kill." "Well, that's yours." [That's *your* explanation, not mine.] "No, that is what they said. And this young sister of ours also said it." Anyway, they have gone to consult some other diviners. But then I completely rejected the idea. I said it was a lie. The brother was sick. Time, his time, had just come, according to my own assessment. I believe it was this AIDS, although I have never seen it. Witchcraft is possible, but in this case, no. My brother died of AIDS.

Silence and Signs

Uncertainty surrounded many deaths. Mutinta numbered the close friends who had died. He was at pains to point out that though their deaths were *assumed* to be from AIDS, he was unaware of any confirmed diagnoses: "All I can say is that a lot more people around, a lot of close friends, have died. Whether it was AIDS or not, well, it's all speculative. I never saw any HIV test results. People die and it is assumed to be AIDS but it is not doctors who have said so."

Where deaths of family members, former classmates, and friends were assumed to be caused by AIDS, this was rarely publicly acknowledged. While there was public silence, there was often private acknowledgment of AIDS, within restricted family circles (though such diagnoses were still open to possible later revision, as, for example, to be the result of a witchcraft attack). Because of the common assumption that most adult deaths from AIDS were the result of "immorality," no one wanted to speak ill of the dead. Discretion and compassion assured silence, or at least circumlocution. Many of those I interviewed suggested to me that speaking directly was not "the Zambian way."[13] Paul's sister, Stella, explained:

> We don't go direct. We go around. It's the way we have been brought up. I think people have always done this in order to try and maintain relationships. Also people don't want to hurt others so much. They are very sensitive, but people are aware. With the dead, people remain very tolerant. There isn't that judgment. When people are very ill, they get short-tempered and sometimes the relatives get fed-up. This is when you find people saying, "You brought it to yourself." Still, most people are very tolerant and they care for their relatives. When there are difficulties, it's mostly because families cannot cope financially.

Sampa spoke of the way people avoided saying someone had died of AIDS, preferring to say "after a long illness." In town where death certificates were required, the cause of death was indicated as malaria, tuberculosis, or meningitis. He thought, beyond the social stigma of AIDS, that relatives were eager to escape; they wished to act compassionately toward the sick:

> You see, no one can say to someone "This is AIDS." No, no, because you see automatically, psychologically, now, you are defeated if you are told like that. You'll say, "I'm sick. I'm sick and I am going to die." So in the end you may just die of depression. From the people I know, a lot of guys who have died and those who are still suffering—they say

they've got TB. But when you see the way they are looking! Ah, well, TB is often HIV-related, isn't it? So no one has ever said to me he was suffering from AIDS, no but, "I was caught with TB." That's all. So you can tell [that it is AIDS]. Some of them are even surviving. They take the TB treatment. They take traditional medicine. They get on well. They put on weight and so for a while they are okay, until the next time.

Zambians became experts at reading the signs that someone was suffering from AIDS. Significant weight loss, especially in conjunction with coughing and skin rashes, was taken as an indication that someone would soon die. Henry's analysis in conversation with me was typical among his peers:

> Do you remember yesterday when we went drinking? There was one gentleman there. You could see it's coming. You can see it in his face. Usually, at first it's the hair. The hair becomes straight. That's usually the first sign. The hair becomes thin and straight and then the loss of weight begins. There is that reluctance to say "This is AIDS," but people know, "That's what this guy has got, that's what this guy has died from." Others will say, "TB," what-and-what. They'll know that it's AIDS but they won't say. It's usually the family members who won't say it's AIDS. They don't want to get to the reality of it and also they want to protect that person. It's often because of the way this disease is transmitted. It seems to be a reflection on their behavior.

However, some of the former students' mothers were ready to name the disease, primarily as a means of warning their other children. Enoch had seen how his older brother, Jones, a house servant, had become sick and he suspected the telltale signs of AIDS. Their mother confirmed his suspicions:

> When I looked at Jones, I said to Anthony [another brother], "Ah, this brother, he's dying." All his symptoms led me to think it was this disease. My mother nursed him. People don't usually say, "This is AIDS," but my mother all along said, "This might be AIDS." She is the one who is always open. And, you know, my mother has known him well. She has seen and known his activities. He had so many women. So she said, "This is AIDS."

A Punishment from God?

Some former students and their wives, in common with many Zambians, concluded that AIDS was divine punishment for human immorality. They maintained that contravening God's law would not go unpunished. However, this was hotly contested by others who argued that God was a loving God; He would not punish people in such a terrible way. Some church leaders in Zambia, Catholic priests among them (see, for example, Dillon-Malone 2004), have attempted to refute the notion that AIDS is a form of divine punishment. Yet, the Catholic Church's public condemnation of condoms implicitly encouraged, wittingly or unwittingly, assumptions about a God who punishes "immorality," that is, "sexual promiscuity," with AIDS.

Strikingly, in conversations and interviews with me about men's extramarital sexual activity, few men, unlike their wives, invoked polygamy as an explanation, indeed as a justification, for the expectation that married men might have other sexual partners. Rather than claiming other partners as simply their due, the majority of men spoke, as in their youth, of "misbehaving" and being "naughty."[14] Some men said they expected God to punish them for their premarital and extramarital sexual activity because the proper place for sex was marriage. Those who understood AIDS as a punishment from God, almost without exception, cited the biblical account of the destruction of Sodom and Gomorrah—which they understood was because of their inhabitants' sexual immorality. No one cited Jesus' compassionate encounter with the woman taken in adultery (John 7: 53–8.11). In fact hardly anyone ever mentioned Jesus. The Old Testament was almost always the sole source for opinions on sexual matters, regardless of church affiliation, though some quoted the Apostle Paul on the duties of husbands and wives. Those Born Again always spoke in terms of "sexual sin," describing it as the worst sin of all. However, they also told me, conversion brought hope.

Elizabeth, Chimbala's widow, had found some consolation in her Pentecostal church. However, she wanted her pastor to speak out directly about HIV/AIDS, to go beyond merely preaching abstinence and faithfulness in marriage. Like other members of her congregation, she believed that God could cure a person suffering from AIDS, if that person had sufficient faith. In her view, AIDS was not a punishment from God. If it were then only "bad people" would be affected, but "innocent women and children" were also suffering and dying. Kangwa rejected the idea that AIDS was some form of divine punishment. Returning to an idea he had first expressed twenty years before, he commented: "It's not a punishment from God. This AIDS is from man. Maybe it was made in a laboratory. Maybe it was made by Americans. Then again, in some ways, it might be the Devil. But then the problem is that God made the Devil and so then God is responsible for the Devil!"

Henry's understanding of God as controller endured in adult life. In 2002, he spoke about family members and close friends who had died from what he assumed to be AIDS-related conditions:

> Last year I lost one of my best friends from St. Antony's, you remember him, Richard. It was AIDS. He got a bit affluent, got married, and then somehow got careless.... Eventually he died of AIDS. Many of my good friends from school and university have died. Some of them, I suspect was from AIDS, others from cancer and one in an accident. The situation is terrible in terms of the fact that you see the numbers of people being buried, especially in towns, especially in Lusaka. And, well, even if my family has not really come to grasp it, well my older brother must have died from this same disease. I say it was AIDS because of his ill-health, the nature of it. If you had seen the condition he was in! Then my cousin, the one I was at university with, I think that is what killed him as well. Then several work colleagues and other friends, more than half a dozen of them.

In Henry's understanding, AIDS could not be a punishment from God, because God did not punish or reward anyone. Henry did not expect to be punished for his own extramarital relationships in which he at times engaged in unprotected sex. He explained:

> I believe there is a God, a controller, controlling everything, but there is no judgment. You cannot judge two people about their lives because they have lived two different lives. Even if we were born on the same day, same minute. You cannot judge me with that person because he has never been me. So where do you get the benchmarks for judging someone? If someone comes in a rage and kills someone, well, that is the way his life has been programmed.

Henry's wife, Pamela, did not think that AIDS was a punishment from God either. She could not recall anyone at her Protestant church preaching on the topic of HIV/AIDS during Sunday services, though she thought it might be discussed during Bible study. Pamela blamed human, especially male, "carelessness":

> If men changed their attitudes, it would make things better. Some women need to change as well. But if AIDS was a punishment from God, then I think he is going to punish all of us. I think it is just a disease. I think it is the carelessness of us people. Some men don't use condoms. I think alcohol has contributed to this.

Simon's brother-in-law had died from what he assumed was AIDS. Simon suspected that his sister might well be HIV-positive, though he had not spoken to her about his fears. He rejected the idea that AIDS was God's punishment. At forty, he doubted that there was any existence after death. There was certainly no judgment:

> I think I take a scientific view. So whatever is that thing that caused life to be as it is—that's what I presume to be God. It's a force, I believe. I don't think I need to believe in all these things like some kind of judgment after death. I don't have the idea of a personal God, no, but of a force, a life force of some kind. (Laughing.) Ah, I don't know where is heaven and hell. I don't know whether there is any life after death. I mean I know matter comes from a number of things and when you die you rot. You become a kind of matter again. It's recycled; it goes into animals and plants. But there is no reincarnation in any sense, no. But then the idea of the soul. I am not sure about the soul. As a scientist, for me, there has to be a number of reasons for things. And, well, I don't see any basis for forming such a theory as the one about the soul. I mean what is the soul? Can anyone define the soul to me? (Laughing.) But well, there is death. When I was ill recently, my girlfriend and my friends came to see me in hospital. I can remember the looks on those faces and I was a bit scared. What was it? Did I have leukemia or what was it? But all the investigations came back negative. I didn't know what was happening. There were times when my mind would just fade off and I just wouldn't know what was happening. And I think you get to that point. When you are so sick and you are aware of it, that sense of being worried, scared of death, the fears. But then as you get more sick, the fear seems to fade also.

Promise did not see God's punishment in Esau's death, though his demise did renew his anxiety that he might be the next one in the family to die of AIDS. Though not a churchgoer, Sampa still described himself as a Catholic. Approaching forty and in poor health, he told me that perhaps Satan (like God, another masculine being) did exist after all. Like several other school contemporaries, he suggested that it was perhaps Satan who had repeatedly "tempted" him to have sex outside marriage, especially when he was drunk. He was unsure whether Satan was responsible for the HIV/AIDS pandemic or whether this was God's punishment for promiscuity. Sampa commented, "Maybe this is just another way of punishing people, that's how I feel. Maybe God has come in another way, actually come to destroy the world." However, these reflections in no way impeded Sampa in his pursuit of extramarital, usually unprotected, sex. Older women in Sampa's family offered other explanations. His maternal grandmother did not think that AIDS was either a new disease or a punishment from God. She and other village elders said that this disease existed a long time ago, even when they themselves were children. In Bemba it was called *ukondoloka* (to grow thin): sufferers became thinner and thinner until they died. There were some people who knew the cure. (See also Mogensen [1997] who records narrative parallels between AIDS and the "traditional" disease, *kahungo*, among the Tonga in Southern Zambia.) Sampa's mother, Margaret, understood AIDS as something that was "in the blood." She offered a commentary on what she judged to be the immorality of her children's generation, and indeed on some of her children, concluding, "It's because of a lack of self-respect." She explained that she had recently "nursed someone at home." That "someone" was her daughter: "She had a cough and diarrhea. At first we thought it was ordinary diarrhea. She became very thin and died. She left one child behind." Margaret understood HIV/AIDS to be God's punishment for sexual immorality: "The prophets said there were many things that would happen as a result of people's bad behavior. It is important to believe in Christ. This disease was prophesied. We were warned, so in this sense, this disease is a punishment. The church is telling us to respect our bodies."

A few other mothers and wives of former students suspected that failure to observe traditional cleansing practices after taboo acts of adultery and abortions lay at the root of the pandemic in Zambia. (See Richards [1982: 36] and Colson [1958: 158] on contrasting accounts of Bemba and Tonga anxieties concerning illness caused by adultery in pre-AIDS times.) Hinfelaar (1994: 166) suggests that in contemporary Zambian society:

> Extramarital liaisons were still feared and regarded as the possible cause of death and misery, especially by the married women. It suited the smart urban males to deny the causative link between *Ncila* (adultery) and the health of his family or the entire community (*Calo*, the land). However, it still lay deep in the psyche of the people, especially the elderly women.

While I found some evidence of this among women, no former student suggested to me that their extramarital relationships might result in illness of any kind through mystical means.

Church Membership

Several men and women claimed that church membership helped them to abstain from extramarital relationships. The churches cited as most supportive in the protection against HIV/AIDS were Pentecostal, although it was among the Catholics that there was the greatest involvement in home-based care groups. Among Pentecostals, AIDS was often described as a form of divine punishment. Former students' membership of Pentecostal churches followed a conversion experience, at times apparently connected with the death of loved ones from AIDS. They cited their conversion experience, together with church requirements regarding prayer and membership of church cells, as forms of assistance that helped them to resist temptation and protect them from exposure to HIV.[15] Several former students' wives were members of Pentecostal congregations. They explained that they believed that if they *were* HIV-positive God would cure them.

It was after the deaths of three siblings within a short space of time from what was assumed to be AIDS that David decided that he had to "get right with God." Before he was officially received into a Pentecostal congregation, David decided that he must tell his wife about a recently ended affair and seek her forgiveness as well as God's. Originally Catholic, at university David had joined a Pentecostal church though he had later "backslid" and stopped attending. He explained his extramarital affair as the consequence of the absence of support from a church group and of his determination to "walk alone." He felt himself, "not so much in slumber," but as if someone had given him "an anaesthetic"—which caused him to fall from his "lofty position." His relationship with his wife had been going through a difficult phase. They had grown apart. When work called him away from home, he met a younger woman. However, David found her increasingly demanding of his time and money. He began to feel like a hypocrite. He explained:

> What I find, when I look back—I find that what really holds me together—the temptations have not gone away, okay? I'm still the same person. But what is it that I am trying to embrace now? That is what has changed my life. I feel like I am a partner with God and I would like to succeed.... So the best deterrent basically, as I might put it, is to have Christ in your heart; it's better than a set of laws or rules governing something.

David's reconversion seemed to put an end to his extramarital affairs, though not to his wife's suspicions of infidelity. Like David, Paul had joined a Pentecostal group at university. He had come to the realization that he had never experienced true conversion. He later drifted away from his church. After several years, many personal disappointments, and the pain of the deaths of his siblings, Paul returned to the church with his wife to be baptized in the Spirit. His surviving siblings, with one exception, became Born Again and attended various Pentecostal ministries. They were convinced that their conversion had been rewarded by prosperity and other signs of God's favor. Harry, Paul's brother, did his best to convert me, encouraging me with the assurance, "It really works!" Paul now committed a substantial amount of his earnings to church coffers by tithing and "giving from the heart" during services. He spent many hours a week in church-related activities, praying at church services early on Saturday mornings and leading a cell group for Bible study and prayer in his neighborhood on Friday evenings, in addition to regular attendance at Sunday service. Paul studied texts downloaded from the Internet sites of popular televangelists such as Benny Hinn. At home the Pentecostal Trinity Broadcasting Network was often the preferred viewing. In his car he listened to Radio Christian Voice or chose from his selection of Pentecostal tapes.

Four of Paul's siblings had died, two of them, his sister Chileshe and his brother Robert, from AIDS-related conditions. Paul had often expressed his anxieties about them to me while they were still alive, but he became even more concerned when they died. Chileshe's husband also died from AIDS within two years of her death. In 2004 Paul's sister, Mary, confirmed her suspicions that she too was HIV-positive. She started antiretroviral therapy in 2005 and responded well to treatment. Paul said that both Robert and Chileshe had been aware that they were dying from AIDS, though Chileshe did not speak about her condition as directly as his brother did. Robert, like Paul, was a university graduate. He had a well-paid job, as did his wife. They had one child. Paul described the course of his brother's illness:

> My brother, he knew what was happening. He went to Chikankata [a Seventh Day Adventist hospital in the south of Zambia, renowned for pioneering home-based care for AIDS patients] at some point; they gave him a very clear prognosis. I don't know whether it catalyzed his death, because shortly after that, he went down very quickly. He lost a lot of weight after that. He had chest problems, TB, Kaposi's sarcoma and so on. I'm saying he knew very well. He would say things like, "You know, I may very well not be here this time next year." So he was getting to that reality.

Paul took a large share in providing for and nursing his brother. He would drive to his home every evening after work to see him.

The family started running out of food. Paul shopped for the few things that Robert felt he could still eat. His brother's long illness and absence from work had several consequences. Robert's employers started to recoup the money they had advanced him in car and education loans. His salary was reduced to almost nothing. Paul paid the house rent. He also took the major share of the very substantial medical expenses, hoping against hope that they could keep his brother alive long enough for a cure to be found. While Paul was ready to try anything, the day finally came when he realized he could no longer manage the costs.

Robert's death was particularly painful to Paul—seeing his brother suffer, watching his life ebbing away. In the last days, Robert was admitted to Lusaka's University Teaching Hospital. By a sad coincidence, most of the hospital staff were on strike. Paul sat at his brother's bedside hour after hour. In the next bed was the emaciated corpse of a young man who had died hours before of AIDS. Because of the strike, no one was prepared to move the body to the hospital mortuary. Later, when Paul went to the mortuary to collect his brother, he was shocked. In death Robert looked much worse to Paul, who observed, "He looked like a little bird, the ribs sticking out, so small, and he had been a big man at some point." He set to work, organizing the funeral. His particular concern was for the embalmers to make his brother look "better" for his mother's sake. He showed them a photograph of his brother when he appeared strong and healthy. In retrospect Paul identified his brother Robert's death as a turning point in his own life, an epiphany, leading him to turn again to God. Paul observed:

> It was a very deep blow for me. He was someone I could share family problems with. And he was my elder brother, so I could always look at myself as number two in line.... As I looked at that body lying there, I knew that my brother wasn't there.... As I sat there, when it finally happened, I heard the women wailing, but I refused to subscribe to the idea that it was finished. I knew that there was a God somewhere. I realized I needed to get right with God.

For the Born Again, deaths from AIDS of close relatives created particular anxieties, concerned as they were for their salvation and convinced that it was now too late to alter their fate. Paul expressed his anxiety about the ultimate fate of his siblings. Dare he hope that even in the last moments of their lives, they had truly accepted Jesus as their Lord and Savior? He chose to hope that, in spite of past sins,

Chileshe and Robert had, in their acknowledgment of God's righteousness, won eternal life in heaven:

> If we fail to make a choice for God, then we may have to face the consequences of that choice when we are living. God doesn't force people; he leaves us free for us to make a choice. From that point of view, I have asked myself, "Do I know what happened to my brother and sister?" I was very scared for my brother, because he only started believing when he was very weak. Well I cannot be sure of a person who has died, unless he says before he dies, "No—I don't believe!" I mean, if he believes in his heart that is even better for me. I don't even need to know. He had indicated that he believed what I was telling him. Then there was a preacher man who went to see him and I think my brother accepted Christ before he died. But basically I stop there because I don't know what decision God made. I mean God is a person like us—who's entitled to his opinion.

While others, especially Seventh Day Adventists, suggested that AIDS might well be a sign that the world was coming to an end, Pentecostals portrayed a more hopeful scenario for the chosen few in this life. While many would be wiped away, a faithful remnant would remain. Paul's sister, Martha, though not speaking explicitly of her siblings, explained that human beings who allowed themselves to be tempted by the Devil were culpable. While it grieved God, they must be punished for their sexual immorality. She described to me how she saw the future:

> People who have died of AIDS have not chosen to die, but they were careless. Even I, if I became careless at some point, I can die. We need to know the season. If the rainy season comes and you haven't brought your umbrella, you will be soaked. So, the season will dictate what you should do. What kind of season are we in? If it is your sexual feelings, you will die. This is a season, which will die. This is a season, which will wipe out anybody who is careless with their lives. God is wiping out the promiscuous. But I think Zambia will pick up. I have dreams of white paper being picked up which means Zambia is picking up. Restoration will come through those who have looked after themselves—the old people and the young generation coming and those who are clean.

Conclusion

For former students of St Antony's and their families the role of "religious beliefs" in their understanding of HIV/AIDS defies any easy summary. Christian missionaries to Zambia have attempted to bring some definition to the figure of God. Apparent missionary certainty has often encountered a huge tolerance for uncertainty among many of those they have sought to convert. Becker and Geissler argue, "Religion allows the possibility of uncertainty, rather than erasing doubts" (2007: 5). God (*Leza/Lesa*) remained "unknowable" and might well be best described, as Colson's Tonga informants maintained, to be like the wind. Former students reminded me, as they had in their youth, that God at times acted "strangely." In the face of the epistemological challenge that the pandemic posed, many former students and their wives contested the portrayals Christian missionaries offered.

Witchcraft that was made to look like AIDS remained available as a possible explanation for someone's death. However, former students rarely resorted to this explanatory discourse. In general, men chose biomedical etiologies over "traditional" ones, figuring themselves as "modern" and "scientific" because of the education they had received. Expert in detecting the early signs of AIDS, out of compassion, they kept silent in the presence of AIDS sufferers and in their talk beyond the family circle. It was left to their mothers to point to the deaths of their children and to spell out the dangers of AIDS. While few men attended church, their prior experience of suffering and misfortune informed their understandings of the HIV/AIDS crisis. Men listened to the various public debates and came to their own conclusions. In general, in this group of former students, non-churchgoing men were no more likely to engage in unprotected extramarital sexual intercourse than others. With the exception of those Born Again, stated religious affiliation, or indeed active membership in a church, was no reliable predictor either of sexual activity in general, or of the use of condoms with wives or extramarital partners. Most wives attended church without their husbands and it was difficult, if not impossible, for them to bring their church's teachings to bear within their own marriages. Where married couples did attend church together, this was mostly, though not exclusively, among Pentecostals. It was within these groups that former students reported experiencing religious conversion and, as a consequence, changing their sexual behavior. They told me that the discipline of regular attendance at church and cell meetings, combined with Bible study, the acknowledgment of their prior sinfulness, and the encouragement of church members sustained them in their decision to forgo extramarital sex.

The pandemic also brought a very particular predicament for those Born Again, left to care for dying family members who, they assumed, had behaved "immorally." Yet I witnessed no condemnation or lack of care and support for those dying from AIDS-related conditions. Wives, unable to communicate their fears to their husbands, might depend upon God to cure them of AIDS. However, men like Paul, while praying that God would intervene, sought the latest biomedical help.

The crisis of AIDS opened up space for the expression of shifting constructions of masculinity within and outside churches. While women bore the main burden of care, some men willingly tended dying siblings, as Promise and Paul demonstrated. While they took no part in domestic chores in the marital home, and only rarely in the care of their children, the suffering of their brothers prompted them to challenge stereotypical "masculine" responses.[16]

8

Responses to Campaigns

Throughout the early years of the new millennium, urban Zambians were bombarded with HIV/AIDS prevention advice and depressing statistics about the scale of the pandemic. Many former students gave a scathing assessment of the campaigns, dismissing the AIDS industry as "just a lot of noise," one ineffective workshop after another in five-star hotels. In Non-Governmental Organization (NGO) and government offices "gender" was on the agenda everywhere, but "changing men" was seen by many Zambians to be an impossible task. One senior civil servant engaged in HIV education and prevention told me, "Ah, Tony, you've lived with us long enough. You know what we African men are like."

More and more people former students knew were dying. It was no longer possible to attend all their funerals because of the frequency of such deaths.[1] Roads in Lusaka and other urban centers were crowded daily with convoys of cars, trucks, and buses in funeral processions. The noise of the traffic was regularly punctured by the wailing of women and the singing of church choirs on their way to the local cemetery.

Few of those interviewed were convinced that the prevention campaigns advising abstinence, faithfulness to one partner, or the use of condoms (ABC) were effective. The majority of former students, their wives, and other family members were heavily critical of the promotion of condoms, describing this as an exhortation to "immorality" and "promiscuity." In 2002 antiretroviral treatment (ART) was only available to wealthy people, businessmen, politicians, and those with connections in Zambia or abroad. None of the men in this study had access to this treatment at that time. The media heralded the imminent rollout of ART to the first 10,000 people, though priority was to be given to medical personnel and other essential workers.

Voluntary Counseling and Testing (VCT) centers were established in urban areas and provincial centers. Campaigns encouraged everyone to learn their HIV status, with the slogan, "It's better to know." Very few of the men and women interviewed at that time for this study agreed.[2] They preferred the "uncertainty" of not having their suspicions about their HIV status confirmed. "What's the point?" former students asked me. They reflected upon past encounters when they had had unprotected sex and assumed the worst. They told me, "The time for me to know will come," that is, when men started to become sick with what had come to be assumed to be AIDS-related illnesses. By the end of 2002 just three out of the thirty former students interviewed had had an HIV test. Edmund and his wife, and Peter and his wife, had had HIV tests immediately before their weddings. Peter said he would recommend that his children have an HIV test before marriage. He explained, "I would even like to see the results of their partners. I wouldn't like any of my children to marry an infected person after I have struggled to bring them up." Simon had been tested several times after a series of illnesses. By 2004 Zambia had 172 VCT sites (Iliffe 2006: 151). A rapid rollout of ART provision followed. By 2006 the Zambian government had eliminated medical fees for patients in need of antiretroviral therapy and over 65,000 people in Zambia were reported to be receiving treatment.[3] At the end of 2007 just over 149,000 people were on ART (2006–2007 Zambia Country Report, submitted to the United Nations General Assembly Special Session on AIDS). By this time five out of the thirty former students had chosen counseling and testing.

Initial reluctance to have an HIV test was not only a consequence of the absence of accessible treatment. Even when antiretroviral therapy started to become available, many Zambians doubted that they could rely on a continuing supply of medication. More importantly, the fear of stigma remained. No former student wanted to be associated with the shame of AIDS, to be accused of "carelessness." Prior to awareness of the pandemic, men known to have multiple sexual partners had been called "champions" by their peers. With the coming of AIDS, men who did not know how to avoid HIV lost their respect. They were censured—in the main—not because they were assumed to have had numerous premarital and extramarital partners, but because they had lacked wisdom. They had not been clever enough to choose with sufficient care, that is, to choose those who were HIV-negative, those who were "clean." They had not demonstrated the cunning of *Kalulu*, the hare, hero of so many Zambian folktales, adept at disentangling himself from seemingly impossible predicaments. However, women continued to bear the brunt of the blame. Men described some women, especially those who appeared to be without husbands or regular partners, as particularly dangerous.[4] With few exceptions, men did not acknowledge that they too might be dangerous to women because of their unprotected sex with multiple, often concurrent, partners.

Several former students were employed to deliver ABC campaigns or in counseling and testing. Yet none of them found it possible always to conduct themselves in accordance with the advice that they offered to others. Paul's sister, Stella, who worked for an NGO, commented from her own experience, "Even people working in the AIDS field can't change their behavior, so what of the others?"[5] Former President Kenneth Kaunda, one of whose sons had died from AIDS in 1987, played a prominent role in ABC campaigns. Kaunda drew upon the commonly held explanation in Zambia that AIDS was the result of sin. Many former students and their wives said it was embarrassing, particularly while watching television with their children, to see him promoting condoms. Kaunda explained that condoms were necessary because of the sinfulness of human beings, what he called "the animal in man."[6]

Continuing Exposure to HIV Risk

Many former students, like their wives, spoke of their anxieties about the consequences their early deaths would have for their children. Warned in their adolescence that their parents might die at any time, now, men, in their turn, pondered the realistic possibility that they might die before their children were old enough to fend for themselves. Promise observed:

> It gives us fear, especially, I would say, people like me. I mean I always pray that I should die after my children have grown. (Laughing.) You know, I have that feeling. I accept that previously, yes, I used to be playful [have multiple partners]. Now if I have that AIDS, if I have AIDS, well, let it come out after the children have grown.

However, Promise continued to "play" with women and to have unprotected intercourse. His prayer was not to be answered. He had a strong sense of being a survivor among childhood friends, and he had resolved not to have extramarital partners from his home village. Promise noted how the land mirrored the failing health of the villagers, as farming production in his home area declined because of the shortage of labor:[7]

> You see, when I am at home in the village, well, I am very conscious—I don't even propose love to anyone there because they say that this

AIDS is more concentrated there. In my home village even now there are a number of people who are sick. Recently, when I have been there—those ladies who I had sex with in the past—a number of them have died. Others are still there, but they are sick. Even some of the elders who used to play a lot [have multiple sexual partners]. In the past the place used to be very lively. We would have a number of Sundowns [beer parties]. It was lively! But now they have stopped cultivating much. Those brewing beer are few because there are few people who have money.

Despite his attempts to be optimistic, Promise at times was filled with foreboding. Like other men, he was quick to lay the blame on women, even though he often spoke frankly to me about his unprotected extramarital sex with different women, as the following extract from one of our 2002 interviews illustrates:

PROMISE: Well, personally, I would say I am free. But, I wouldn't say much on that one. Maybe, ah, maybe, if I have had that problem [be HIV-positive], then it must have started three or four years ago. I mean, that is AIDS. If I have that AIDS, then I must have had it three or four years. I mean I used to go out with a certain lady some time back. Ah, you know, going out with these ladies, they are also movious. They have some other men also. They have some other men, especially when you are not there. Maybe when you are at home with your wife, then they have other men. But of late I have tried very hard. I mean I have stayed almost two years without going out with anyone else—except those ladies I told you about. I mean before that I had these other two ladies—and that's where I doubt if they were very safe. I doubt. Because I used to go out with them openly [without using condoms].
TONY: Why was that?
PROMISE: Ah, well, with one of them, I knew her for a long time. I knew her in 1992—that's when I first knew her, first had sex with her. She was somehow steady, according to the way I took her. When I first started going out with her, there were no men that I had heard of going out with her. Then later we parted. Then I went to live in the north. By chance she also moved there and I met her again. Now, I had that mentality that she was still ok. So we started again. It's later that I discovered, ah, you can never know with these ladies. I mean she can be going out [having sex] with other men. But then I was already going out with her. Anyway, I stopped. I mean there were a number of men who had gone out with her.

Like other former students, Promise made a distinction between women whom he described as "prostitutes" and other women he had sex with. In his experience, the "prostitutes" generally insisted on condoms. He contrasted their insistence with other women, "especially ladies in the villages" where "it's up to you, the man. You decide whether you use a condom or not." At Promise's favorite nightclub, the security guards facilitated sexual encounters. For a small fee of 5,000 kwacha, they spread sheets of cardboard on the ground outside the club. In 2002, for a "fast round," the women charged 15,000 kwacha (around U.S. $3), or 20,000 kwacha (around U.S. $4) with a condom. Taking a woman for the night cost much more and involved booking a taxi to take her to a hotel room or a friend's house.

In Sampa's view, the future in Zambia was bleak because of AIDS. He recognized that he and his children might well die in the pandemic:

> As for the future in Zambia very many people, very many are going to die of AIDS because (laughing) even these kids we are producing— Yah!—well, we don't know, maybe they are HIV-positive. People say, there was some survey, by 2010, these young children who are nine or ten, they will have died of AIDS because of their fathers. Maybe I could be one of them, I don't know.

Despite what he had learned about HIV transmission, like many former students, he still indulged his preference for unprotected extramarital sex. Sampa acknowledged the risks he was taking, but argued that it was simply "natural" for a man to desire multiple partners and to want to "go live." As he and most of his school contemporaries had insisted in their younger years, he claimed to be able to discriminate between those women likely to be carrying the HIV virus and those who were not. His judgment was based on what he saw of a woman's behavior. Like others among his school contemporaries, he acknowledged the influence of alcohol, but he also blamed the Devil, as the following interview extract indicates:

> TONY: Why would you take such risks? You know others who have died of AIDS, don't you?
> SAMPA: Yes, many, very many! (Laughing.) Ah (laughing), Mr. Simpson, that question is a very, very difficult one to answer. These days, even me, when I see a girl, well, the first thing I think is, "Maybe she has got AIDS." But then, okay, you talk, you talk and then you are on top of her. But maybe she says, "Can you put on a condom?" So, psychologically, you feel, "No, this girl is clean. If she can tell me to put on a condom, that means that she always uses condoms" and so (laughing) as for me, I will go direct [have unprotected sex]. You

carry on; you just do it. That's why it is better for someone to get married. Then, every time you want it, you just think of your wife. Actually, you are right, it's a big risk. Sometimes it's just alcohol. When you are drunk, you look for a girl. You look at her and you just feel to have sex with her. I mean for most men these two—drink and a girl—they go together. And then, even when you are not drunk, the feeling you have for a girl, you are not even thinking about AIDS. With me it has happened. You sleep with a girl and after the game is finished, [you think] "But why did I have to do that?" After I am satisfied and I no longer have that feeling—"No, why did I have to do this? (Laughing.) Why? Why?" I don't know. Maybe Satan is in between us. Maybe it's Satan. Really it might be Satan. Otherwise, why do that?

Sampa appeared to waver between hope and fatalism. He repeated often-heard remarks such as "*Ubu bulwele bwaikala pacakulya*" ("This illness is in that which is eaten.") and "AIDS is a disease and diseases are for human beings." But still, he had restrained himself because of AIDS, he claimed:

Ah, you know, Tony, this issue, look Tony, I wouldn't cheat you. Everybody is worried about it. Ah, it's a question of time. I don't know how I'll put it.... But sometimes, ah, I mean not that I have actually given up my life. No! Look, I mean, using my position, well, I could have done it [had sex] with any girl I felt like. I could have had a lot of ladies, but I actually avoided them because of this same issue, this AIDS.

Catholic Teaching

For Catholics the use of any form of contraception directly contravened their church's teaching, which condemned condoms both as a method of contraception and as a means of HIV/AIDS prevention.[8] However, no self-identified Catholic former student gave this as an explanation for not using condoms. (There was a noticeable public silence on the part of church leaders in Zambia about contraceptive pills and injections.) Margaret, Sampa's fifty-seven-year-old Catholic mother, spoke angrily against the promotion of condoms that, she said, were spreading AIDS. "Is this condom new?" she asked rhetorically. Margaret regretted that parents' abstinence advice to children was contradicted by their own extramarital sexual activity. Despite giving birth to her first child, Sampa, out of wedlock at the age of fifteen, like others of her generation, she claimed that in her youth she had had no sexual experience.

One argument apparently supported by many Catholic Church leaders in Zambia was that the HIV virus was small enough to pass through condoms, thus rendering them ineffective. Some former students, and not only Catholics, agreed, though this added to their anxieties. David, for example, formerly Catholic and now Born Again, worried about a past affair: "How small is the virus? How much smaller is it than the sperm or the bacteria? Could it have passed through the condom? And in any case, if there had been a bit of abrasion on the rubber, how difficult it would be to determine if the virus had flown across."

Aware of the numbers of people they suspected had died, or were dying, from AIDS-related conditions, most respondents agreed that condoms were ineffective against HIV. "The condom is a deceiver," they explained. This conclusion chimed well with most men's extreme reluctance to forego pleasure and intimacy by using condoms. Former students and their wives, regardless of religious denomination, accused local Catholic priests of undermining the church's message about sexual abstinence outside marriage because of their own sexual activity. (See Setel [1999: 178] on "mischievous priests" in Tanzania.) Sampa, nominally a Catholic, was sympathetic; sexual abstinence was abnormal for any human being. However, Paul, formerly Catholic and now Born Again, criticized Catholic priests for their failure to lead the celibate life they had promised. Henry, a self-identified Catholic though not a churchgoer, explained that he had been discouraged by the behavior of Zambian priests: "I'm a Catholic. I believe in what is preached but I don't necessarily accept what is done—like this celibacy. You see what these Zambian priests do? The complete opposite! I mean the man has taken a vow of celibacy and he's having sex with women, even having children. We know a lot of these guys."

Several men spoke about the number of Zambian Catholic priests dying from what were assumed to be AIDS-related conditions. They pointed to the wealth that priests had at their disposal, a house, a car, domestic workers, the leisure and freedom to pursue affairs with women.

What to Tell the Children?

Though there were a number of exceptions, most former students and their wives argued that the only message to be given to their children was that of abstinence.

Malama's wife, Eileen, favored the abstinence message. She knew twelve-year-old girls who had boyfriends. She thought she should speak to her girls and her husband should speak to the boys. Eileen had started to teach her twelve-year-old daughter about sex. She considered herself fortunate that she had a "very frank and open" woman neighbor who helped her in this task. She summarized their advice: "We tell the girl to be careful about razor blades at school. We tell her that if she has sex with a boy she will develop sores all over her body."

A few former students and their wives took a pragmatic approach. Although Elizabeth, Chimbala's widow, had not told her youngest son that his father was dead, she was determined that he should know the dangers of HIV infection and the means to avoid it:

> Children should be taught about AIDS. My children, like my son who's six—he asks questions and I just tell him the truth. I asked him whether he had seen a condom and he said he had. I explained to him what it is and what it does. At his [Seventh Day Adventist] school, they are being told that condoms are bad. My view is that if one cannot possibly abstain, then they must use a condom.

Sampa was adamant that his son should be taught to use condoms in premarital sex. He maintained this view, even though he had been unable to follow this advice in his own sexual activity, whether premarital or extramarital, and his boast of never having caused a pregnancy out of wedlock was contradicted by what he had told me:

> It can be very difficult. However, when my first son is fifteen, that's when you can tell him to be using condoms, one, to prevent pregnancies and two, obviously, the AIDS issue. So you just have to tell him, "Be careful! You are still going to school. Me, I've never impregnated anybody in my life-time." Sometimes you may need to be frank with them, "Me, I used to sleep with a lot of ladies, but I knew what I was doing. Also you should be told by your teacher. A girl should know her cycle. So, don't have sex without a condom!"

Henry hoped that he would be able to be open with his children about sex and the dangers of HIV/AIDS. He thought abstinence messages were unrealistic. He favored the promotion of condoms, though, like Sampa, he was unable to follow this advice in his own extramarital affairs:

> Well, I cannot say to them, "Never have sex!" I mean that is fallacious. It's just not possible. Besides I am not always there to see what this person is doing. My daughter has sex education at school, so she knows

the disadvantages of having sex without protection. She must know. I must tell her frankly. I think, in these times you don't leave it to chance. I will advise my children, "If you have to have sex, then you have to have it with protection—always!"

Pamela, Henry's wife, was pleased that anti-AIDS campaigns were being transmitted in Zambian languages on the radio. However, she was against the promotion of condoms because she thought they encouraged promiscuity. She judged that the appropriate age for children to begin to learn about AIDS was twelve. In her view, they should only be taught abstinence. With her daughter she was ready to use scare tactics: "When there is an advert about AIDS on television, I have asked my daughter what's being talked about. At school she's been given the information and pamphlets on AIDS. I add a little more information. I have taught her indirectly and I have scared her that if she goes with a man she will be out of school."

Mutinta was among those men who considered most campaigns, especially workshops in hotels and game lodges, a misuse of available funds. In his view, information should be disseminated in bars and workplaces and at people's homes, door-to-door. He considered it was much too late to focus on abstinence. What was needed was more intensive promotion of condoms, despite opposition from many church leaders. Mutale, his wife, expressed very similar views, adding that cartoons should be used to teach young children.

THE HIV TEST: BETTER TO KNOW?

Several men and women said they supported the idea of testing in principle, but had no immediate plans to discover their status. Reluctance to have a test was most often based upon the expectation of having their fears of an HIV-positive status confirmed. The fear of being stigmatized was uppermost in many minds. However, there was also the widely held conviction that a positive diagnosis would hasten their deaths. They said that if they discovered themselves to be HIV-positive, they would be "psychologically defeated" and, as a consequence, would "die sooner." They found it difficult to imagine how, in the language of the awareness campaigns, they might find a way to "live positively." Besides, in the contemporary uncertainties of life in Zambia, many former students explained, they might well "die another death." For many men the limits of a particular construction of masculinity were revealed. They told me that they were not "brave enough" to hear what they assumed would be a death sentence. Darius explained that, *in principle*, he thought it was good for everyone to know their status. If both partners were HIV-positive, then in his view, there would be no need for them to use condoms. However, he was too afraid to have the test:

> I am scared. I might go through what I went through when I had gonorrhea. Then I was always thinking that since I had gonorrhea then I had AIDS as well. I went through torture. I even grew thin. I was scared. I wouldn't [didn't] even have any appetite. I was scared. I feel I might go through that. I am scared of AIDS. Unfortunately we are not keen to know our status, but if the AIDS is already in us then we are going to pay for our history.

Promise's continuing good health persuaded him that for the time being there was no urgent need to know his HIV status. Reflecting on past "misbehavior," he explained:

> Personally, it has frightened me. I wouldn't even want to have a test. (Laughing.) I mean, if I happen to be found positive, I might be *very* worried! No, I have just thought no, I can't have a test. No. Ah, I mean if you knew [that you were HIV-positive], ah, you would be doing things in a very retrogressive way. Ah, you'll be thinking, "Though I do this, any time I might die." I mean me, here, if I knew I had AIDS, ah, even me, here, no I wouldn't have come for further training. I mean I would have thought, "I'm just wasting my time. Any time I might leave [die]." And you can be beaten psychologically, and then you die sooner. It's true. Better you remain without knowing. Well, in one way or another, it makes me get worried. Because at times, when I recall my life, I also think, "Maybe I am also one of them who is going to have this. I have done this before." But, well, maybe the time is not yet ripe to have that stuff exposed, otherwise, well, you see, I always have that feeling.

Fear was only part of the problem. Very few husbands and wives discussed whether to have an HIV test. Former students anticipated that a wife would react unsympathetically to a husband's positive diagnosis. Wives did not insist on their husbands having a test, despite fears about their extramarital activities. In 2002, Paul's sister, Stella, suggested that most men were reluctant to discover their HIV status because of their extramarital activity. She knew of both husbands and wives who were aware that they were HIV-positive and who continued to have unprotected sex without informing their partner of their HIV status. She repeatedly complained about the lack of communication between partners, especially about women's submissiveness:

> In the African tradition, this is entrenched. How I wish women could say to their husbands, "Condom or no sex!" I remember a couple who came for an AIDS test. The woman came out negative but the man proved positive. When I asked the woman what she thought about using condoms, she said, "It's up to my husband." It just shows how submissive we are.

Simon's work included HIV testing and counseling. He exemplified the attitudes and feelings of most former students:

> A lot of people do not want to know whether they have it or not. And, if anything, they know who is at risk, and they know that they have been at risk. And for them they think, "Well, what's the point in having a test? I already have it. I am dying anyway, so what is the point of curtailing my social life?"[9] It is not necessarily that they want to go out and infect many more, but they just want to carry on with their life, the way it has been. They know that they have been exposed and they feel, well, it is not going to make any difference. They class themselves as positive. But I can understand in a way. Well, they probably do not want to know because it is very probable that they do have the virus. I mean they won't be mentally strong to take it in and so they are going to be more or less depressed rather than anything. So then they think, well, the depression will cause them to go down quickly.

In 2002 Kangwa told me that he had decided he would not have an HIV test. He had recently suffered from TB and it had taken him a long time to recover. He recalled his past sexual activity and feared the worst, though he rarely explicitly expressed his apprehension. Because of his significant weight loss, he knew others assumed that he was dying from AIDS:

> As you see, I am thin and it's a problem. It's a problem being thin in Zambia today because people suspect you have AIDS when you are thin. I wouldn't have a test. Look, the nature of my work, especially in the past—going into rural areas, working there, having relationships there. You see, at that time we thought this AIDS was found in town, it wasn't something you would find in the village, no. There was that belief that there was no AIDS in the rural areas. But, when I think of maybe five or six relationships where I was having unprotected sex, no, no, I wouldn't have a test. There is no point. No, look, Mr. Simpson,

I don't think it matters. Even if I had had only three relationships, if one of those was with someone with AIDS, then I am already HIV-positive. There is no point in having a test. It won't help, no. Look, I know this. When I am happy, I am healthy. But when I start to worry, that's when I get sick. I won't have a test. Those years I was exposed, especially up to about 1996. You know whether you were exposed to HIV or not. I won't have a test and, among all my friends, not one of us will have a test. There is no point. There is no medicine. There is no help.

Kangwa wondered what would happen if his wife, who had been very sick, became aware of his status, were he to have a test that should prove positive. It was difficult for me to believe that she had not suspected AIDS as the cause of their ill-health. However, they had never discussed having a test, as Kangwa explained:

We don't discuss such things, not directly anyway. We have never discussed having a test. And my wife, ok, she is thin, she has lost a lot of weight but she is healthier than I am. As for me, well, I had a problem with TB but that is over now. I am back at work. I get a lot of problems with my throat, sore throat, but that's all, though I am not as bouncy as I used to be.

Enoch, formerly an HIV/AIDS counselor, had chosen not to have a test himself. He estimated that he had had around thirty sexual partners. He had rarely used condoms and, like other former students, spoke of the threat women posed in the transmission of HIV without acknowledging that men might pose a threat to women. Enoch highlighted his fears of the recriminations from his wife that he imagined would follow a positive test result:

I haven't had a test myself even though I used to be an HIV counselor! I've never thought about having a test (laughing). But as for now, well, I am okay. There is no big illness over me, but, well, I could be HIV-positive. But you know, considering how many partners that you've had in the past with those ladies. Well, now out of all those relationships, well, one of those women could have given you HIV. But if you are married it becomes very difficult. What can you do? It would be very difficult to use a condom every time you have sex. All along you have been having unprotected sex. Now, how do you change? Your partner will be suspicious. You know how life is. You usually point fingers, "You are the one!" "No, you are the one!" I don't know whether my wife has had a test. I don't think so. If she has, she has never told me. We have never discussed it.

David said that in a recent extramarital affair his greatest fear had been that he might make his girlfriend pregnant. He said he had been complacent about the risk of AIDS, commenting, "The question of AIDS disappears if you get very close to someone, because you don't think of them in that objective manner." In 2002, now Born Again, he explained his reluctance to be tested for HIV. Like several other men, he claimed it was not the possible knowledge that he was HIV-positive that he feared most, but rather what he foresaw were the insurmountable problems that he would face in communicating such a diagnosis to his wife:

> Well, how can I put it? (Long pause.) I would like to have a test but, ah, I don't have the inclination to have one somehow. I do not feel the urge to go and have a test. Maybe, if it was just to clear my mind, maybe I would like to have one, to get that assurance that I am ok. As to the consequences, I would be cheating if I said I wouldn't be afraid of finding out if I have this disease which is terminal in nature—or potentially terminal. I think that I would be afraid initially, but I think that's where it would end. But I think I'd love to know.... I've said I thought I've made a mistake. But it also gives me a greater sense of responsibility for it. I think, if I went and found out [that I was HIV-positive], then I'd say, "Well, this is my situation." Purely statistically, mathematically speaking, it would help me to plan my life better, maybe you know, should I start taking medicine? Should I start planning for my departure, for the sake of the kids and my wife? But it is more than that. It's the issues that relate to my wife. How do I tell her? And how does she react to that? It does get very complicated from that point of view, from the point of view of human relationships. Maybe someone who is single can face it in a simpler manner because he may not be with those partners.

David realized that even his albeit slight suspicions about his HIV status posed a problem in that he continued to have unprotected intercourse with his wife, potentially putting her at risk. He could find no way to resolve the conundrum. After long discussion, he commented to me:

> Well, basically, it's an issue that I would prefer to forget about. Taking action on the other side of it would mean acknowledging it every day—which becomes quite a load. And in that case, the only option would be to find out so that you either remove that load or you find out for sure that you need to carry it. So it's a little bit of a difficult decision. On face value, when you look at all the facts, it looks like going for an AIDS test would be the best option; but I've never really sat down to consider my

situation. But as you talk to people and as you come across situations, sometimes you just feel that pinch, ah, that lady [former sexual partner] (laughing), should I contact her, find out how she's doing?

Before his readmission to the Pentecostal church, David decided that true repentance required that he tell his wife about his recent affair.[10] His marriage survived, though with difficulties. He realized that he had underestimated her reaction in his urgent desire to remedy the situation. He observed:

> I found out there was still consequences to be faced. You get forgiven at the end of the day; nevertheless, you still face the consequences. And the consequences continue. Well, I think I wouldn't be able to say much for my wife. But I get the feeling that she knows that I am a changed person but maybe her ability to trust me completely, maybe, has been defeated by that whole episode. So I need to earn the trust all over again and I don't know how I can do that.

Paul's sister, Martha, was Born Again. When I visited her, I would sometimes have to wait until she had finished her prayers. She prayed aloud in her bedroom, often speaking in tongues, shouting in a rough manly voice, so unlike her own soft spoken, gentle tones. She spoke on many occasions about the problem of AIDS and of her own experience, explaining that she had had only one sexual partner. A single mother with two young children, Martha said she would like to have an HIV test. To date she had not done so, even though tests were readily available. She was confident that she was HIV-negative. Even if the test result was positive, she explained that God could cure her. Only faith was required. She assured me, "With God nothing is impossible. We have heard of testimonies of people who had full-blown AIDS but got cured. Cry for healing and repent!"

Henry said he had never seriously considered having an HIV test, though he was the only former student to say he was confident that he could cope with a positive result. His wife, aware of some of Henry's extramarital affairs, was reluctant to have an HIV test. Like many other women and men, Pamela feared that a positive diagnosis would shorten her life. Many wives were reluctant to discuss in any detail their fears of contracting the HIV virus from their husbands, though their anxiety was clear. Malama's wife, Eileen, aware of her husband's past infidelities, worried about his current behavior but preferred not to be tested:

> In the past I heard a lot of things about my husband. This time it seems to be different, but the truth is no one should trust her husband

because men are difficult. AIDS is in the homes among married people and not only among prostitutes. I feel happy at the moment. However, one never knows what the future has. I might be happy here, when in fact I have the virus.

Agatha said she was ready to have an HIV test, if her husband, Hambayi, would agree to have one too. But he would not. He said he saw no need. While Hambayi told me he trusted his wife, he was aware that Agatha had certain misgivings about him and his behavior. She did not trust him, but she had never told him so directly because, she explained, she had no evidence to confirm her suspicions about him. In his untrustworthiness, Agatha thought her husband was just like other men. She feared that he might infect her with the HIV virus but was unable to discuss this with him. She dreaded what might happen to her children, should she die from AIDS before they had reached an age when they could fend for themselves. Agatha believed it was better for everyone to know their HIV status: "Once you are told that you are HIV-positive, you are also told how to look after yourself. AIDS is causing many problems. For instance, if I were to die, my children would suffer. My mother is old. She is sixty. My sister is poor."

Simon had been troubled by ill-health recently, including an episode of TB. He repeatedly suffered from flu-like symptoms and feelings of exhaustion. He had had several HIV tests, all of which had proved negative. Simon attributed his lassitude and weakened immunity to stress and overwork. His family, especially his mother, however, suspected the worst; he explained: "Even my family thought, 'Ah, HIV!' Well, with my mum I wasn't so surprised. I mean she sees people dying of TB all the time. Anyway, when she came to see me, I said, 'Look I've had the test,' but I don't think she believed me."

Sampa's Illness

Sampa's reluctance to end the "uncertainty" about his HIV status exemplified many former students' approach to the predicament they found themselves in. Many men appeared to be in a state of denial. It seemed almost that anything was preferable to being given an HIV-positive diagnosis, which was generally understood to be a death sentence. The absence of communication between husbands and wives isolated partners and increased anxieties.

Despite two years of poor health, Sampa repeatedly postponed having an HIV test. He had cause to suspect that AIDS might well be at the root of his ill-health, but was not prepared to have his suspicions confirmed. His wife, Ruth, often worried about the possibility of Sampa infecting her. She regularly expressed her anxieties to female members of her family but not to Sampa. She had had an HIV test at an antenatal clinic before her marriage and had tried on several occasions, without success, to persuade Sampa to have a test as well. He had repeatedly promised her that he would have one, but had not done so. Toward the end of 2002 Sampa's health worsened alarmingly. Added to this, Ruth left him for another man. Sampa lost weight, had no appetite, felt increasingly weak, and was troubled by a persistent cough. After a course of antibiotics, the cough had gone away—only to return worse than ever. I suggested that he might have a medical check-up and a test for tuberculosis. After a while, and with no improvement in his health, Sampa agreed. He was prepared to receive a diagnosis of TB. He was well aware that most people associated TB with AIDS. Indeed he had the recent example of the death of his cousin's husband but Sampa was not ready to face the prospect of a test that might confirm that he was HIV-positive. He preferred to attribute his ill-health to depression following the departure of his wife and his struggle to gain custody of his children or perhaps a combination of depression and some yet-to-be-diagnosed sickness—but not AIDS. Several of his friends had TB and were receiving treatment. If it was TB, Sampa reckoned, early awareness would increase his prospects of recovery, before, as he put it, his lungs were "completely eaten away." His ambivalence about his illness was evident in the way he spoke about his impending medical check-up, using language familiar in Zambia in HIV/AIDS campaigns: "Ah, well, it's better you know. And then you start. Then you are living positively. You see, it's very bad if, when you are down completely, that's when they find you with TB. Those people, they don't survive." As he grew weaker, Sampa began to discuss with me the possibility of having an HIV test. When I asked him whether he suspected AIDS, after a long reflective pause, his reply was ambiguous:

> Well, I wouldn't suspect that one, but I am just thinking of that. No, no, not AIDS as such, but chest, chest, TB. It's okay to go. Maybe, actually I *will* have an HIV test. This time I am so brave. (Laughing.) Because I have nothing to lose (laughing)—I don't have a wife! So it's better you know your position. You reduce this thing of drinking beers. Doing what-and-what, you reduce.

Sampa rejected my suggestion that he might have an HIV test at one of the "New Start" centers at the minimal cost of 1,500 kwacha.

He preferred to have a check-up at a private clinic. One of his friends had regular check-ups there, paid for by his employers; he offered Sampa his place for free. It was not simply a question of cost. Like other former students, Sampa believed that staff in the private sector were more likely to respect confidentiality. Several men spoke of "childish" doctors and nurses at government hospitals who gossiped about those discovered to be HIV-positive.

Sampa's mood darkened as his strength deserted him. He did not have the energy to carry a bucket of water from the well to bathe. His stomach was swollen. He had pain on the right side of his body—in his right lung, he thought. He had grown thin and was so weak that he needed to be carried to the outside toilet. One gray, windy day in the cold season, I found him sitting outside the partly finished house he shared with family members and paying lodgers. As I approached the house, Sampa turned to his nephew and cousin, two young boys, and said, "Here comes the right person to bury me!" He seemed convinced that it was the end. His relatives took him first to a nearby clinic. Here tests on his sputum were inconclusive. They brought him home again but on the advice of a nurse, who was a family friend, they took him to the main hospital in the town where he had a chest X-ray. On my next visit, Sampa brought out his X-ray to show me and pointed to a shadow on his right lung. The possibility of HIV/AIDS came uppermost in his mind, when Sampa was finally diagnosed to be suffering from tuberculosis, though he did not lose all hope, as he explained:

> At the hospital they said that they had found some fluids in the right lung. So I asked the doctor if this had anything to do with my swollen stomach and he said, "No, actually, this is TB. So we will put you on TB treatment."... There at the hospital they didn't give me anything. They just took the X-ray. But I brought it here and the people at the clinic here put me on TB treatment. I forced them to explain to me why it was like that. Because, (laughing) if you are following me quite well, Tony, you know that I used to play with [have sex with] a lot of girls. So I believed that ah, this is now AIDS. So I asked the very person who was taking the X-ray, "Could this be AIDS or what-have-you?" So he laughed at me, "No, don't talk about AIDS. This is just TB. It has been there. Even a long time ago, people used to suffer from TB. But, however, there are certain cases where with this TB, with some people it's very serious. Now, that's when you can say, ah, they are suffering from AIDS. So, ah, we don't know. You will see it for yourself. If you don't respond to the medicines, then maybe." But according to me, well, I think I have responded to the

medicines. You can see the results. You can see (pointing to his forehead) these pimples. They told me that this is a sign that I am responding well. So when I came to the clinic, I asked them the same question. They said, "No, don't be worried. If it is AIDS, you will see yourself." Still, at first, I was convinced I was dying actually, especially these diseases like TB. Once you discover that you are suffering from TB, well, people associate it with AIDS. They feel, maybe, you are in the same line. But as of now, now that I have been taught about it, it's not always that when you are suffering from TB that you automatically are suffering from AIDS. There is a lot of TB in the world. It doesn't mean automatically that you have got AIDS, especially here in Africa.

Sampa's preferred state of uncertainty about his HIV status continued. He told me what he had learnt in weekly lessons at the nearby clinic and how he had been encouraged to "live positively":

SAMPA: They say, even with AIDS, sometimes you can live positively. And then with good diet, you can be okay. People live up to ten or fifteen years. They are HIV-positive. So I believe that it is better that you know.... They give us lessons about AIDS. And they tell us, "You should be using condoms." Ah! (laughing) Tony, you know about me in terms of condoms, don't you? (laughing). It's not my favorite, actually (laughing). We have classes every Wednesday—me and these other patients who are also suffering from TB. They tell us what to eat. They tell us to refrain from sex. I mean they tell us to stop having sex with these ladies.
TONY: Completely?
SAMPA: Ah, Tony! No! (laughing). Ah, that's not possible. Ah, no! I was emphasizing on that question, "Are you saying stop *completely*?" So the nurse laughed. She said, "No, those who are married, no, once in a while it's not bad, but use a condom." But again, the problem there is that, well, as you know, when having sex, well, you should have power, energy. And you lose a lot of proteins. That's why maybe they want to stop us from having sex. You lose proteins. You know, sperms are proteins in nature.

Sampa's anxiety about losing proteins and energy was short-lived. Following a chance meeting with one of his former wife's friends, he arranged to bring her back to his room for sex. He explained that, despite his aversion toward condoms, on this occasion he used them because in his convalescent state he was anxious to avoid contracting a sexually transmitted infection (HIV did not apparently figure in his equation) and equally importantly he had no wish to make the woman pregnant. In common with the majority of former students, Sampa considered women a threat to his health but he did not in the first instance think that he might pose a risk to women:

SAMPA: That was my first time for me to have sex with her. But I used condoms. As you know I am sick. And I mean I could have some grazes on my penis so it's not—well, I mean I could have some sores—and these ladies, ah, you know, they can have some diseases, so I used a condom. I didn't want to take any risks. I mean I didn't want to get some disease from her, or maybe even impregnate her. Such things, I didn't want.

TONY: And what about you? You could give something to her, couldn't you?

SAMPA: (long pause) It's true. It's true. It's not fair. But as for me, ah, I'm okay. I mean it's not something to do with AIDS (laughing). No, this is just natural TB.

TONY: Well, I'm just saying you might give her something. I mean the way you put it, it sounds like you think she might give you something, but you don't seem to say that you could give her something.

SAMPA: (long pause) Okay, okay, it's possible! It's possible! It's true. Even me, I could give her something.

Sampa's health gradually improved. He carefully adhered to the tuberculosis treatment regime and faithfully attended the weekly sessions at the local clinic. He scoured the local market daily for the best fruit and vegetables that he could afford. Though he had expressed his anxiety that he might be starting with full-blown AIDS, he once more postponed having an HIV test: "What I have decided is that any time, maybe after three or four months, I want to go for an HIV test. I mean actually there is no need for me to be afraid of whatever. I just have to go for an HIV test." His indecision, however, would continue.

CONCLUSION

No former student explicitly said that the prevention campaigns had caused him to change his sexual conduct. Some of the men, a minority, were not engaged in extramarital affairs. Yet, with the exception of those Born Again, this seemed to reflect the pattern of their sexual activity since their youth—and not because of the campaigns. The majority of former students and their wives questioned the morality of condom promotion. Many doubted that condoms could prevent HIV infection. Instead, they supported the increasing emphasis on abstinence in prevention programs such as those funded by the American President's Fund that fitted well with Christian discourse about sex and their notions of respectability.[11] While there were some dissenting voices, most parents considered that abstinence was the only message that their children should hear—this despite many men's sexual careers having commenced at an early age. Additionally, men and women considered the numerous deaths of family and friends from what were assumed to be AIDS-related illnesses as evidence of the ineffectiveness of condoms. Few attributed these deaths to men's refusal to use condoms, or to the difficulties entailed in ensuring appropriate and *consistent* condom use. Most former students continued to have unprotected sex both inside and outside their marriage. Many remained concerned about the condom's capacity to impede their achievement of speedy ejaculation, especially in sex with extramarital partners where a man's "sexual strength," his essential manliness, needed to be definitively demonstrated. The gaze of the peer group was never far away. Men continued to consider extramarital partners as likely sources of HIV infection. They tried to reduce the risk by avoiding "dead" (AIDS-infected) women, and regretted when, especially under the influence of alcohol, or the "excitement" of money, they considered that they had failed to protect themselves—as much by their choice of partner as by the omission to use condoms.

Many former students assumed they were HIV-positive, but chose to try as far as possible to "forget" their worries, to suspend their anxieties about their health and their children's future. They anticipated the time when illness would confirm their fears. The limits of manliness were reached, as most men said they were too afraid to have the test. Unwilling to address their own worst fears, former students felt secure in the knowledge that, as "tradition" dictated, their wives would not openly challenge them about their HIV status. Wives did not confront husbands with their extramarital affairs. Despite many wives' apprehensions that their husbands might well give them HIV, most felt trapped, unable to speak to their husbands about this.[12] Some women placed their trust in God to protect and cure them. They were convinced He would touch them.

Through 2005 and 2006 antiretroviral therapy gradually began to be more and more available in urban areas. In spite of this, most former students continued to procrastinate about having an HIV test, thereby avoiding the illocutionary act of a positive diagnosis and the associated stigma. Were they to test HIV-positive, husbands could not imagine how they might discuss this with their wives, though most thought they could tell their mothers. The absence of trust and of communication between the majority of married partners extended to this most difficult of issues. Uncertainty remained the pragmatically preferred state of being. While many former students told me of their anxiety for their married sisters' health, few explicitly expressed this concern about their wives. They appeared genuinely surprised by my insistence of the threat they posed to women.

Former students' continuing exposure to risk of HIV infection (or reinfection) has several possible explanations. Their reluctance to use condoms was not simply a reckless disregard based upon condoms' capacity to "tax" men's pleasure. Many spoke of how condoms prevented intimacy. They explained that they felt they had not "really met" a woman if they did not have "live" sex. Because of their assumed, but unacknowledged, HIV-positive status, they decided that there was nothing to be gained by practicing "safe sex," especially with their wives for whom, they judged, the introduction of condoms would merely increase their well-founded suspicions.

The campaign messages that former students and their families heard rarely went beyond ABC advice and exhortations to take an HIV test. There was no space for the exploration of the terrain in which sexual encounters within and outside marriage were embedded. The existing gender order—men's power and men's claims to power—generally went unchallenged. The campaigns failed to address the contexts of Zambians' lives where women felt unable to protect themselves from the risk of infection from their husbands and where men were rarely challenged about their preference for multiple partners, "skin-to-skin," "tight-and-dry" sexual intercourse.

Most former students saw huge obstacles to responding in the ways that campaigns urged. This was not because they did not accept the biomedical discourse in which they were framed. Rather, it was because they were unwilling to accept the consequences that attending to the messages would entail—surrendering some of the "patriarchal dividend," foregoing some sexual pleasure and intimacy, and having to acknowledge their "misbehavior," their "carelessness." They imagined many difficulties, not least among them depression and the speedy death that they would face should they discover, beyond doubt, that they were HIV-positive. It was better not to "know." The widespread absence of communication between most husbands and wives—and between men and their girlfriends—about the risk of AIDS created a wall of silence. Men might imagine the virus incubating in their bodies, but the majority decided it was better to keep their fears in check, by not addressing them, until such time when physical changes made it obvious that they were succumbing to the pandemic. Who knew what would happen in the interim? They might die another death.

9

CONCLUSION

"I have tracked my game; now I have speared my meat."
—Bemba bridegroom's song (Richards 1982: 106)

What might we learn from the lives of this cohort of mission students who came to manhood in the shadow of AIDS? And how might this contribute to the transformation of gender relations and the greater involvement of men in efforts to combat the pandemic? Former students' early lessons in gender and sex—both at home and at school— provided them with particular models of how to act in the world like "real men." They had to be strong, silent, and keep their emotions to themselves. From an early age, the men in this study felt under pressure to demonstrate a risky kind of masculinity to themselves, and to others, especially other boys. As young children, and as pupils at primary and secondary school, they learned sex and gender through the body.[1] Their apprenticeship in desire through their embodied experience produced in them certain corporeal styles (Butler 1990: 139). They rejected the example of their celibate missionary teachers. With few exceptions, from an early age, most students took an eager part in the play of sex. Despite anxieties about their competence, they enjoyed sensual pleasure unsullied by the fear of AIDS. To be sexually active was simply to be human.

Most boys and young men endeavored to perform an acceptable version of Zambian masculinity. Exceptions, like Peter, recognized that they fell far short of this. Peter thought of himself as "lame," crying when distressed, lacking the courage to approach girls for sex, experiencing his first sexual intercourse only at marriage. Some young men, such as Paul, Simon, and Mutinta, tried to resist the hegemonic version of masculinity that entailed multiple sexual partners. This was, in part, they explained, because of shyness and their desire to succeed academically, but also because they questioned the validity of this construction. As young adults they became acutely aware of the dangers and injustice to women that this entailed. Most former students, however, strove in youth and adulthood to demonstrate their manliness through repeated sexual conquest. Their continuing socialization as adults led them to reiterate particular performances of masculinity that put them and those they had unprotected sexual intercourse with at greater risk of HIV infection.

Despite different emphases in the histories of masculinities among ethnic groups in Zambia, most former students felt that they were required to show themselves as conquerors, hunters of women, as in the Bemba bridegroom's song.[2] They exhibited many aspects of male gender power and yet, I argue, they were in turn overpowered by ideologies of masculinity, of male heterosexuality, that rendered them, and their sexual partners, vulnerable to AIDS. Undoubtedly, they benefited from the "patriarchal dividend," but the emotional and physical costs have been overwhelming; some have paid with their lives.[3] Local constructions of masculinity remained salient for former students as they pondered whether to have an HIV test. Apart from Peter, Edmund, and Simon, others remained extremely reluctant to attend Voluntary Counseling and Testing Centers. Illness would eventually drive three more of them to have a test. Despite Kangwa's earlier pessimism, with the increasing availability of antiretroviral therapy (ART), he relented in his determination not to discover his HIV status. In mid-2005 he and his wife were both found to be HIV-positive. They began ART immediately and two years later were continuing to respond well. In 2005, Sampa suffered a further bout of TB. He still hesitated about whether to have a test. He had started a new relationship and planned to marry. However, he began to suspect that his return to ill-health might be caused by his new partner. She was a Satanist, he concluded; she had to kill him in order to demonstrate her commitment to Satan's cause. Giants appeared to Sampa in his bedroom at night, trying to persuade him to join the Satanists too by killing his son. He adamantly refused, assuring me that he would rather die. He lost more weight and suffered from recurring nightmares. Even in the daytime, Sampa could see an old crone perched on his shoulder. She pursued him everywhere he went, even to the pit latrine. Growing weaker and weaker, Sampa finally resolved to have an HIV test. He was diagnosed HIV-positive. Instead of commencing ART, he enrolled on a program to investigate the efficacy of the treatments of traditional healers and spent several months secluded with other participants in the trials. By mid-2007 Sampa had regained his weight and his strength and had not started ART. He began a new relationship and fathered a child who was born

HIV-negative. Illness drove Promise to have a test. He discovered he was HIV-positive shortly before his death from AIDS. Susan, his wife, discovered she was HIV-positive and started treatment. By mid-2007, none of the other men in this study had had an HIV test. David, Paul, and Henry remained in apparently good health and continued to postpone having a test, though David's wife was tested at an antenatal clinic prior to the birth of their son. Darius had bouts of ill-health and suffered considerable weight loss, but explained he remained too afraid to discover whether his illness might be AIDS-related. Many former students felt ill-prepared to deal with the consequences that such knowledge would bring. There was a limit to what manliness could demand of them.

Berger et al. have argued, "But men must do more than admit their complicity in patriarchy; they must begin to rethink the very boundaries that shape and define what it means to be a man" (1995: 7). The pandemic has brought a new urgency to the need to redefine and redesign gender relationships. This work must start at an early age both in the home and at school. While the school may not be the key influence in the formation of masculinities, schooling has been recognized as "the most powerful influence across the board, and in some cases and some situations it is decisive. It may also be the most strategic, in the sense the education system is the setting where an open debate about the democratization of gender relations is most likely to happen, and can gain some purchase on practice" (Connell 2000: 147).[4] This has enormous potential when young men and women are mutually engaged, breaking the isolation often imposed by their respective gender projects.[5] Process Drama is one means by which boys and men may begin to rethink and refigure what it means to be a man when faced with the demands of social justice in the time of AIDS.

Process Drama

My work in Zambian schools with Brian Heap, a Process Drama expert, has demonstrated that process drama can be a useful tool in the furtherance of such democratization that necessarily entails addressing the dynamics of gender power.[6] Employing the language and the techniques of drama has a number of precedents in the social sciences. Victor Turner drew upon performance as he developed theories of social dramas and an "anthropology of experience," emphasizing throughout his work the transformative potential of ritual (1974; Turner and Bruner 1986). Erving Goffman drew upon theatrics in his analysis of notions of self, self-presentation, and how the self might become stigmatized (1959, 1963). Their interests in drama led them to participate in experimental theatre workshops with Richard Schechner (1985). Using drama in the context of HIV/AIDS has particular relevance if we build upon Butler's insights into the manner in which gender is produced through repeated performance. Changing gender relations will necessarily entail learning to perform gender in novel ways.

To promote HIV/AIDS competence, that is, the ability to live a healthy life in the time of AIDS, the social, political, and economic terrain of people's lives, "the social matrix of sexuality" (Connell 2000: 126), must be taken into account.[7] Process drama offers an avenue to engage young men and women both in analyzing the political economy of HIV/AIDS and in devising personal solutions to survive the crisis.[8] Analyzing life contexts inevitably entails examining how gender is learned, understood, and performed. This is a necessary prelude to understanding how individuals perceive and act in sexual encounters that are always socially embedded. Process drama is created not for a watching audience but for the benefit of the participants themselves. They are the ones who, together with the teacher or facilitator, make meaning *for themselves*. Employing Freirian techniques of "learning from below" (Freire 1983), the participants in this whole-group drama process "write" their own play as the narrative and tensions of their drama unfold in time and space through action, reaction, and interaction. The aim is to develop a dramatic response to situations and materials from a range of perspectives. (See Bowell and Heap 2001.) Heathcote describes drama as a "progressing art" and comments, "By using this truthful artificial environment students can face up to emotional, affective, 'people' responses before finally having to practice in society" (1984: 197).[9] Bruner suggests that every culture maintains institutions such as storytelling and theatre which have "'forum-like' features...ways of exploring possible worlds" (1986: 123) that offer participants an active role as participants. Process drama is a type of ritual passage where a shift into the subjunctive mood is facilitated. Turner developed Van Gennep's delineation of the structure of rites of passage, drawing attention to the indeterminate, "subjunctive" mood of the liminal state, which may be a period of intense creativity. Turner noted when "historical life fails to make cultural sense performative and cultural drama may have the task of *poiesis*, that is, of remaking cultural sense" (Turner 1982: 87). The crisis of AIDS presents the challenge of how to make sense of it and how to survive it. Goffman in his frame analysis also alerted us to the creative potential of the subjunctive, to use activity "as a model upon which to work transformations for fun, deception, experiment, rehearsal, dream, fantasy, ritual, demonstration, analysis and charity" (1974: 56). Turner and Goffman both noted the importance of "frame" in everyday life. Heathcote, drawing upon Goffman's work, uses the term to describe the element that gives tension to drama. In process drama, "frame" situates the participants in relation to the unfolding action and gives them a sense of *investment*. Taking a role means imagining that you are someone else in a fictional context and exploring a situation through that person's eyes. The role may be a group role embracing all the participants and the facilitator's main task may be identifying that role and thus helping to focus the group on the issues and tasks of the drama. Within the group, there always lies scope for individual difference. The role is nothing without the frame—the tension giver.

Among the many concerns of Zambian secondary school pupils in 2002 was the problem of intergenerational communication on sexual matters and how to decide what conduct would be appropriate for themselves in the time of HIV/AIDS. They demonstrated in various ways a keen awareness of the prevailing gender order, revealed, for example, in the still images they produced of the "typical" Zambian family. In one coeducational day school in Lusaka,[10] after lively negotiation class members agreed to arrange the family with father and mother standing together and the children arranged according to their order of birth. The facilitator then invited various members of the class to come out to the front of the class to rearrange the family members in the still image according to what they thought would be most appropriate. Once they had rearranged the family members in the still image, the facilitator asked them to explain their decisions.

The girl who had taken the role of mother stepped out of role to rearrange the family. She put the first-born daughter and the last-born daughter together, commenting, "The last born is always liked by the first born." She put the boys according to birth order after the parents, followed by the girls, the oldest daughter being positioned at the end of the line after the last-born child and explained, "The oldest daughter has big responsibilities for her brothers and sisters. She gives advice to them. She behaves like a parent. She is the mother when the mother is not around." The girl/mother then explained why the boys were arranged close to the parents, "Sons are given more respect than daughters." The facilitator asked the class to explain and was first greeted with a response in chorus of "It's tradition!" Then a girl explained, "The second born, that's the oldest son, will become the father if the father dies." Another girl commented, "Girls will not inherit property. So girls are put at the end." A third girl added, "If she is a widow, she no longer has power. So she's put at the end."

No boy took a lead role in explaining the way the family was configured. However, relative status according to gender, gender-specific responsibilities and power was immediately revealed by consensus in the class. Males were positioned "higher" than females, and hence afforded greater importance, and were placed by female students before females who were acknowledged to be the main caregivers. Although pupils readily explained "proper" conduct by resorting to explanations such as "It's tradition," in hot-seating sequences they demonstrated awareness of other possible ways of behaving and a conviction that change was possible. Pupils questioned the father of the fictitious family being portrayed who expressed gender-typical sentiments about not feeling any great responsibility for the direct care of his young son, whom the class had named Chico:

> BRIAN (FACILITATOR) TO CLASS: Now this is your chance to question members of the family.
> GIRL TO CHICO'S FATHER: Do you think you will play a big role in looking after Chico?
> FATHER: No. I think most of the time the child will be with the mother.
> BOY: Will you play with the child?
> FATHER: No, not really.
> BOY: Are you going to teach the child how to behave?
> FATHER: It's too early.
> BRIAN: So it looks like you think Chico's father has little to do here.
> *(Class members now question Chico's mother.)*
> GIRL: What are you going to do to make sure that your child remains healthy?
> MOTHER: Go to the antenatal clinic.
> GIRL: I have a suggestion for Chico's father. You should help around the house, change his napkins and play with the baby. At least you should do that.
> GIRL: The father should start to develop a relationship with Chico even when Chico is young.

The girls in the class were clearly not satisfied with the answers given by the father in the drama, in particular to questions asked by boys. They quickly offered advice to the father that contradicted the portrayal of the "traditional" Zambian family they had earlier articulated. The drama appeared to be assisting the students in the interrogation of their own notions of family, gender, status, and power. It would be wrong to suggest that the boys produced only stereotypically "hypermasculine" responses. They demonstrated considerable sensitivity in their suggestions of how best to care for Chico during the prenatal phase. A striking instance of young men's readiness to take up nurturing roles was observed across several sites. In a drama created by pupils at other schools about stigma and an orphaned older sibling's dilemma about how to provide care for an HIV infant, the HIV-positive baby was signed into the room by the facilitator by folding a piece of cloth (*citenge*) into the shape of an infant and handing the "baby" to the student who had agreed to represent the infant's teenage sibling. Each boy who received the "baby" spontaneously and without any apparent self-consciousness or desire to "play up" to the group began to comfort the infant by rocking her/him gently in his arms.

Process drama may lead to further debate and discussion. As among the former students of St. Antony's and their wives, many of the pupil's parents expressed strong disapproval of "sex education," judging it to be simply encouragement to have sex and an opportunity to promote condoms. While there was some murmuring of dissent when abstinence was proposed by some class members as the best form of protection from the HIV virus within the drama, a number of pupils asserted that this was indeed the best solution overall. The majority in the class did not want their parents to talk to them about using condoms. This, in their view, would be tantamount to encouraging sexual license. On the issue of condom use, there was a range of opinion:

> BOY: I wouldn't like my parents to give me advice about using condoms.
> BOY: No, you have to abstain. Using condoms will mean I will be committing a sin against God.
> GIRL: Abstinence is the best way. Condoms are not 100% safe.
> GIRL: We are still young. We should not be using condoms. Abstinence is best. It's in the Bible...
> BOY: If you have been advised to use condoms by your parents, then they are not stopping you. The parents could be encouraging you.
> GIRL: O.K. Abstinence is the best thing, but you have friends. They also influence you. Now condoms, O.K., they are not 100% safe but still, we teenagers, we have that mind to experiment. So we should use condoms.
> BOY: I disagree. Fornication is a sin. God says, "Don't do it."

GIRL: People sin. Parents should give us a choice! If you haven't abstained, then you should use condoms. Now, without condoms I could get AIDS and how is that going to help?
BOY: No, that's not good.
BOY: No.
GIRL: Most of the time parents, mothers, they say, "You are going to get pregnant." They don't talk about HIV/AIDS. But some friends advise taking the pill, but that won't prevent me from getting AIDS.

Clearly the students shifted out of role for the purposes of this discussion, referring to "my parents" or stating "we are still young." A broad range of opinion was expressed within the group. The process drama experience had not brought the participants another message about HIV/AIDS but had, rather, opened up opportunities for the participants to explain their knowledge to themselves and others. The process drama practitioner facilitated a shift into the subjunctive exploration of alternatives. No naïve claim is made here that the drama in itself produces a sudden change in attitude and behavior or that this might be confidently assessed. Clearly, in tandem with personal change, radical transformations are required in the political, economic, and ideological structures of the gender order.[11] However, process drama promotes an affective engagement with the human dimensions of situations—an essential stage in efforts to encourage safe behavior and to promote compassion. Reid highlights the importance of creating empathy in HIV prevention. She observes: "Empathy creates the possibility of a way forward. For empathy allows the coming together across barriers of difference and creates the possibility of responses of respect and inclusion.... It is a moral skill which enables the recognition and valuing of others. But the valuing of others essentially involves caring for self" (1997b: 11–12).

In all schools where the pilot study was conducted, cross-gendered role-taking was a marked feature. At times the frame chosen by the facilitator dictated this and thought-tracking inevitably drew at least some members of the class into a cross-gendered role. This offered considerable scope for the articulation and appreciation of other-gender perspectives. In contrast to top-down approaches, process drama creates an arena for participants to bring their own concerns to bear in the dramas they actively create. In process dramas young Zambians demonstrated how relationships within the family impact upon their understandings of themselves as engendered sexual beings and revealed how gender may be subject to rearticulation and change. There is the potential to break down the wall of silence and pretence that often exists between men and women around sexual risk-taking. In the fictions they compose, participants may explore and reflect upon the sometimes harsh realities of their everyday lives—but in the safe space that process drama can create. In this way boys and men may become aware of the diversity of masculinities (Connell 2000: 226).

Masculinity as Performance

In their youth, few students at St. Antony's had appeared secure in their sense of themselves as men. At secondary school, it was common with many boys and young men in Zambia, when they felt shy or particularly anxious, especially in the presence of older men or strangers, to shield or cup their genitals with their left hand. Their action suggested both a desire to comfort themselves in their unease but, more crucially, albeit unconsciously, to protect their deep sense of vulnerability. Savran highlights the anxieties that surround masculinity. He observes that "a gendered identity, on account of its contingency, is of all identifications the one most subject to intense social pressures, the most anxiety-ridden, the most consistently imbricated in social, political and economic negotiations" (Savran 1998: 8). If *white* masculine identity in the United States is, as has been argued, "built around an anxiety of insufficiency" (DiPiero 2002: 9), how much greater might be the anxieties that surround black masculinities in postcolonial Africa, globally implicated, as they have been in Zambia, in large-scale political, economic, and social forces that have wrought radical transformations in personal life?

On the face of it, many former students of St. Antony's had the upper hand socially, politically, and economically in gender relations. Yet, while they exhibited the requisite manly bravado in the public presentation of themselves, many men were acutely aware of the artifice entailed in the heterosexual performance of masculinity that involved the sexual conquest of women. Most former students figured their extramarital (usually unprotected) sexual intercourse as "misbehavior" and described themselves as "naughty" and "mischievous," seeming to evade acknowledging the dangers of HIV risk by using terms normally associated with childlike, if not childish, behavior. Wives might say that "Men are children" and "Men are difficult," but they felt unable to challenge their husbands about their extramarital sexual encounters and the risks that these posed for them. Most former students seemed imprisoned within the demands of particular constructions of masculinity, the fragility of which was revealed in the repeated performance of what was judged by male peers to be "proper manly" performance. They were anxious to be seen publicly to live up to the ideal of the "real man," while they were ready privately to acknowledge, at least to me, the pretence that this entailed. Confronting men about this charade remains a matter of urgency if gender relations are to be transformed. (See Baylies and Bujra 2000: 179.) This necessarily entails the need for men to gain a deeper understanding of themselves, especially at the emotional level.

Despite recent rapid social change, former students' marriages echoed many of the complexities of marital relationships in earlier times. The ethnographies of marriage rituals and of rural married life by Audrey Richards and Elizabeth Colson are redolent with images of male power and instances where etiquette required the wife to subordinate herself to her husband. Yet these accounts also reveal the ambiguities in gender relations, the give-and-take of marriage. Colson records that among the Plateau Tonga the wife accepted the role of servant to the husband. She would bring his water for washing and drinking. She cooked and tasted his food and drink to demonstrate that she had no designs on his life. The husband rarely fetched and carried for his wife, "but a woman thinks nothing of unceremoniously dumping the baby into her husband's lap with instructions to mind it while she occupies herself elsewhere" (1958: 141). Richards's account illustrates similar apparent contradictions in Bemba gender relations. She noted men's apparent power in many aspects of day-to-day living: "Menfolk are dominant in Bemba society. Women used to greet men kneeling and they still do so on formal occasions today. Men receive the best of the food.... They speak first in family matters.... Women calmly accept that their husbands will beat them 'when they are young and their hearts get hot quickly' " (1982: 50).

In her account of the Bemba initiation rituals, *chisungu*, that she observed in 1931, Richards drew attention to the ways in which the virility of the bridegroom was emphasized. Toward the end of the ritual, the bridegroom was required to enter the hut in which the girl had been instructed, carrying with him a bow and arrow. Aiming carefully, each bridegroom had to shoot one arrow into a round mark on the soft whitewash of the wall above the head of his bride-to-be. Richards describes the marriage ceremony that followed as "a test of his procreative powers; he must give a sign of his potency by throwing a burning brand out of the house on his marriage night" (1982: 150). Richards highlights the paradoxical contrast between the depiction of the bridegroom's role in the *chisungu* and his position in daily life: "In village affairs he must be submissive and quiet, as befits a stranger. He works under the orders of his in-laws and only gradually wins his position as head of his own family. In the *chisungu*, he appears as a roaring lion, a lion-killer, a crocodile, a hunter, a warrior and a chief" (1982: 158). Richards notes the contradictions that find expression in *chisungu* and in everyday life "between the masterful male and the submissive son-in-law, between the secure married woman backed by her own relatives and the submissive kneeling wife." She suggests that such contradictions might be regarded "as an extreme expression of the dilemma of a matrilineal society in which men are dominant but the line goes through woman" (1982: 50).

The recent history of Zambia demonstrates the mutability in constructions of gender and in gender relations themselves. Many young Bemba men, once described in their marital role as isolated strangers in their wife's village, would become, under colonialism and increasing globalization, part of a mission-educated elite, "breadwinners" in urban households. With men's formal education and economic power, in urban areas it was women rather than men who most needed to be married. Urban living has brought its own tensions in relations between men and women. Economic decline and the enrichment of a few (mostly men) has given yet another twist to gender relations, especially for those former students of St. Antony's who struggle to provide for their families.

From early life, most of the men who have featured in this study were entrained into particular performances of masculinity—performances that entailed pretence. In the shadow of AIDS, it is important to recognize that these performances of masculinity can be transformed. Men in Zambia, as elsewhere, need to be disabused of the illusion of an abiding, essential male-gendered self (Butler 1990: 140). If men are prepared to acknowledge the deep sense of insecurity and fragility that underlies, indeed often drives, their manly swagger, the prevailing gender order might be radically transformed. Then the long-wave event[12] of the HIV/AIDS pandemic might still hold liberatory potential for women (Baylies and Bujra 2000: 197) *and* for men.

Writing of Bemba marriage in the 1930s, Richards noted how custom required that Bemba wives carried loads while husbands walked unencumbered. Yet, Richards observed how this was merely part of the performance of Bemba masculinity. Men would actually help their wives with the loads, when they thought they would be unobserved: "I have met husbands helping their wives with some heavy task, such as carrying wood, but they felt it necessary to do in secret and to hand back the load to the woman on entering the outskirts of the village. This was part of an established behavior pattern and universally accepted" (1969: 93).

It is high time for men in Zambia, and elsewhere, to be challenged to take an equal share in the burden that AIDS has brought. Some men have already taken up this challenge and many more, I am convinced, will be ready to do so.

Notes

Chapter 1

1. Students explained that the term derived from the fact that new boys often cried for their mothers—like chicks separated from the mother hen (Simpson 2003: 123).
2. There was, and remains, a wide age range of pupils at primary and secondary schools in Zambia. Various factors, among them poverty, influence the age at which a child begins schooling, and events often intervene causing pupils to interrupt their formal education or to repeat grades. In the 1980s young men beginning their secondary education might be as young as thirteen and as old as eighteen.
3. See Iliffe (2006) for an account of the spread of AIDS in the region.
4. In the mid-1980s, U.S. Census Bureau Population Division, Washington, estimated HIV-1 seroprevalence among pregnant women in Lusaka to be 8%. By the end of 2003 the UNAIDS/WHO estimate of people in Zambia living with HIV/AIDS put the adult rate (15–49 yrs) at 16.5%, with a low estimate of 13.5 and a high estimate of 20%.
5. http://data.unaids.org/pub/EPISlides/2007/2007_epiupdate_en.pdf.
6. See Turshen (1998) for the impact of World Bank reforms on the promotion of the privatization of health care and the subsequent decline in access to African health services.
7. The 2002 research, entitled "Men and Masculinities in the fight against HIV/AIDS in Zambia" (R00023493), was funded by a fellowship from the Economic and Social Research Council, United Kingdom. I am grateful to two local assistants, Dixter Kaluba and Chitalu Mumba, for interviewing school contemporaries of the original cohort and wives of former students, and for their insightful discussion of the data.
8. There are seventy-two, some say seventy-three, ethnic groups in Zambia. Bemba-speaking people are originally from the north of the country and Tonga-speaking people are from the south. St. Antony's success drew students from far and wide and this was reflected in the ethnic composition of the student population.
9. The rate of exchange fluctuated during 2002, but averaged about 4,500 kwacha to the U.S. dollar.

10. For reviews of anthropological HIV/AIDS research, see Akeroyd (1997); Farmer (1997); Schoepf (2001); and Parker (2001). For a review of anthropological research on masculinity, see Gutmann (1997).
11. See Baylies and Bujra (2000: 179).
12. A monograph that overcomes this shortcoming, though it does not discuss sexuality, is Werbner (1991).
13. In his account of the lives of Ghanaian men, Miescher chooses to focus on what he terms a "narrative self," highlighting self-presentation tailored to specific audiences (2005: 202).
14. I am grateful to Penny Harvey who addressed the committee's concerns in my absence, pointing out to them the crucial role of establishing relationships in anthropological fieldwork.
15. See Jacobson-Widding (2000) for similar descriptions of a boy's relationship with his father and mother and of the ideal male personality type among Shona-speaking Manyika of eastern Zimbabwe.
16. Two women did leave their husbands for other men, though in neither instance did they cite their fear of AIDS in their decision.
17. The terms "African" and "European" are used in Zambia as synonyms for "black" and "white," respectively.

CHAPTER 2

1. See Connell (1995: 122) on the need to go beyond the mother and father in any analysis of how boys learn to be men. For an autobiographical account of boyhood in Zimbabwe, see Shire (1994).
2. Fortes (1974) suggests that the birth of the first-born, especially the first-born son, marking as it does a father's irreversible transition to parenthood draws his particular attention to the child in a relationship that entails ambivalence and ambiguity.
3. See Richards (1939: 140) and Colson (1958: 240).
4. See Ritchie (1943), Powdermaker (1962), and Epstein (1981, 1992). No former student expressed any memory of being weaned.
5. A recent report (Muvandi et al. n.d.), based upon surveys, questionnaires, and focus group discussions conducted in and around Ndola, on the Zambian Copperbelt concluded that men and women in all age groups were "somewhat reluctant" to accept the concept of gender equality.
6. For a discussion of the relationship between corporal punishment and claims of "ownership" in Nigeria, see Last (2000).
7. While some caution is needed with respondents using English as a second language (Last 2000: 367), the severity of many of the beatings described is evident.
8. Campbell (1992) has explored the manner in which boys in Natal first learn within the family to view violence as a socially sanctioned means of resolving conflict. Walker reports numerous examples of South African men remembering their father's violence when growing up, "of

either witnessing their mothers being beaten or fearing the regular and violent beatings they received themselves" (2005: 7). For a recent discussion of fatherhood in South Africa, see Richter and Morrell (2006). In surveys, 40% of Zambian women have reported being regularly physically abused (Heise et al. 1994). Comparable figures for other African countries were Kenya, 42%, Tanzania, 60%, Uganda, 46%.

9. This taboo suggested a general fear of incest between a father and daughter. Affluent Zambians who hugged "big" (post-puberty) daughters were often criticized by former students for adopting, in *this* instance, dubious "European manners."

10. Though some of this respectful behavior might have been occasioned by my presence, I observed such conduct both from a distance and by chance; it was a regular feature in some homes.

11. Colson (2000) offers cogent arguments for the increase in witchcraft accusations by children against Tonga fathers.

Chapter 3

1. See Richards (1969) and Colson (1958) for descriptions of such play among Bemba and Tonga children. Pattman and Chege report six-year-old Zambian children speaking of their sexual experiences, "almost in the same breath as play" (2003: 100). They were, however, conscious that their parents would disapprove.

2. Men learnt later that women were taught at initiation how to "dance in bed" and, although to adopt the missionary position, to be anything but docile.

3. Delius and Glaser (2002) argue that there was a degree of intergenerational communication on sexual issues in precolonial African societies in Southern Africa and that the communication gap between South African youth and their parents is a recent phenomenon.

4. Dover (2001: 108) reports the same warning given to Goba boys.

5. Rasing (1995: 52) records this teaching in girls' initiation rites in a Copperbelt Roman Catholic community. See also Rasing (2001).

6. The Zambian Demographic Health Survey for 2001–2002 (Central Statistical Office of Zambia 2003) reports the median age for what it terms "sexual debut" as around seventeen years for both boys and girls. The survey notes that approximately 18% of girls and 27% of boys aged fifteen to nineteen have had sex before the age of fifteen.

7. For similar observations on the links between excellence in sports and schoolwork and the ability to attract girlfriends in South Africa, see Niehaus (2000).

8. Mair (1953: 81) notes how marriage between cross-cousins (children of a brother and sister) had been the ideal among matrilineal peoples in Central Africa and that Bemba parents of either a boy or a girl were entitled to claim a relative in this category as a mate for their child. Richards (1969: 24) and Colson (1958) comment on the earlier preferential

cross-cousin marriages among the Bemba and the Tonga, though by the 1950s this type of marriage had lost favor among the latter.
9. See also Simpson (2003: 23–24).
10. Young men had told me that kissing, especially on the mouth, was a "European" practice, formerly unknown in Zambia. Some said it was unhygienic. Many students said that Africans who witnessed scenes of men and women kissing found their sexual appetites quickly aroused. Films that contained such scenes were often greeted with roars of laughter by the student body at St. Antony's. For some years after Independence, kissing, like violence, was censored on Zambian television and in films.
11. As teenagers and again in middle age, men stressed to me that human beings had sex but it was God who decided whether their intercourse would result in a child.
12. Such views parallel those recorded by Richards among earlier generations of Bemba people: "Both men and women will describe what they find physically attractive in the opposite sex. But in the choice of a wife they do not seem to be guided by the ideal of romantic love as it is understood in present day middle-class Europe or America" (1969: 22).
13. Following the deaths of many family members and friends from AIDS, Edmund later became a strong advocate of condoms.
14. Ages of both boys and girls at primary school, even in the same grade, varied widely. In grade six or grade seven ages might range from twelve or thirteen to as much as seventeen or eighteen.
15. Current policy is that pregnant schoolgirls are allowed to return to school after giving birth.
16. This terminology is widely reported in Africa. For Zambia, see Dover (2001), Dählback et al. (2003), and Rasing (2004: 4); for Kenya see Ahlberg et al. (2001).
17. See Segal (1990) for the inherent potential in heterosexual performance for a man to experience a sense of failure, ineptness, and confusion. See Holland et al. (1998) for a similar focus on male performance among young men in British cities.
18. Dählback et al. (2003: 60) report similar expectations from adolescents in focus group discussions conducted in urban Zambia.
19. See Richards (1969), Colson (1958), and Dover (2005) for Bemba, Tonga, and Goba perceptions, respectively. Colson observes that among the Plateau Tonga young children engaged in masturbation as part of their sexual experimentation: "Small boys and girls masturbate without any notice being taken of it by older people, and small boys occasionally engage in mutual masturbation in public" (1958: 272). Richards (1969: 16, note 2) mentions evidence of mutual masturbation as an indication of "homosexual" activity among boys. Both Richards (1969: 16) and Colson (1958) describe young girls meeting in small groups to practice the custom of enlarging the labia by stretching, as a preparation for full adult sex life. Richards observes that some of the young girls in these groups joined up in pairs and referred to each other as husband and

wife. On the practice of stretching the labia as part of sex education in Zimbabwe, see Jeater (1993: 24). See also Dover (2001: 97) for a discussion of prohibitions on masturbation in Africa.
20. In Genesis (Chapter 38: 7–9), God kills Onan because he "spilt his seed upon the ground." Onan did this to prevent Tamar, Onan's brother Er's widow, from becoming pregnant. Several Christian traditions, particularly the Catholic, have cited Onan's fate as a warning against what they considered the sinful practice of masturbation or *coitus interruptus* (withdrawal).
21. See Douglas (1966).
22. Hambayi is showing me respect by his apology, demonstrating that talk about sex between young people and those judged to be of their parents' generation were generally considered inappropriate.
23. See Laqueur (2003) for a cultural history of masturbation in the West.
24. See Laumann and Gagnon (1995) for "circle jerks" elsewhere.

Chapter 4

1. In the 1970s and early 1980s there were places in secondary schools for less than 30% of pupils who completed the seven years of primary education. Though secondary school place provision has increased with the establishment of Basic Schools (grades one to nine), at the end of 2006 there were grade eight places for only just over 50% of those pupils completing grade seven. Those children who "fail" to win a place in grade eight are often referred to as "drop-outs," though in public discussion in Zambia they have been more correctly identified as "squeeze-outs." See Serpell (1993: 11).
2. The number of children men had, or anticipated having, was on the whole far fewer than their fathers had had. Wives were still of childbearing age in 2002. Most married couples had either two or three children. In 2002 there were exceptions. Joshua and Sarah had five children. Hambayi and Agatha had four, though they had another child in 2004 despite the couple's joint resolve not to have any more children. By 2005 Paul and Matilda had four children.
3. By the time Promise had reached the age of forty there had been nineteen such women, the latest being a woman half his father's age.
4. For example, in Bemba the verb "to marry" is *ukuupa* (active voice) for men and *ukuupwa* (passive voice) "to be married" for women.
5. While "well-built" is intended to mean, "have a 'good' figure," students did not find slim girls attractive. In addition, as the symptoms of AIDS became more apparent, slim young women were often suspected of having "Slim"—one of the early terms used for AIDS in Zambia, as elsewhere in Africa.
6. In recent years AIDS has taken a disproportionately heavy toll among teachers. See Kelly (2000).

7. Sampa's mother, Margaret, here makes no distinction between *lobola* and *nsalamu*. *Nsalamu* is the first token payment in marriage negotiations that the man offers to a woman's family through a go-between (in Bemba, *bashibukombe*) as a statement of his wish to marry her. *Lobola* is the substantial payment.
8. "Movious" initially describes someone who constantly moves from place to place. However, it is also applied to those who have multiple sexual partners.
9. The importance of being a father for Sampa was demonstrated in our own relationship. Initially, Sampa had led me to believe that his second wife's children were both his, though I later discovered that she had had her first child with another man.
10. Formerly menstruation and *cisungu* instruction immediately preceded marriage among the Bemba. Richards (1982) offers the classic detailed account of this instruction. See also Corbeil (1982), and for contemporary marriage instruction on the Zambian Copperbelt, see Rasing (1995). Colson notes that among the Plateau Tonga a girl's puberty rite, which included an extended period of seclusion known as *ku-vundika* (from the verb "to place to ripen"), "lacks many of the educational features which enrich the puberty rites of tribes such as the Bemba" (Colson 1958: 281).
11. See Richards (1982). Colson (Personal Communication 2007) notes the difficulties a fieldworker encounters in attempting to enquire into husbands' and wives' sexual relations, a topic that brides are instructed as belonging to "the secrets of the house"—not to be divulged to outsiders.
12. "Sex with a husband during menstruation is unthinkable" (Richards 1982: 32). However, Colson reported, "The Tonga do not fear sex with a menstruating woman" (1958: 139).
13. On older women's attempts to police younger women in rural Tanzania for the benefit of men as husbands, see Bujra (2000: 131).
14. For discussions of this practice elsewhere see Burke (1996: 29) for Zimbabwe, Parikh (2005: 134) for Uganda, and Kaspin (1996: 83) for Malawi.
15. Richards observed:

> To remove the dangers due to sex intercourse a special ceremony is required and this is one which can only be performed by a legally married couple.... At marriage each girl is presented by her paternal aunt with a miniature pot about two and a half inches in diameter which must be guarded with the utmost secrecy. With this the purification rite is carried out. It is filled with water and placed on the fire, man and wife each holding the rim. Water from the pot is then poured by the wife on to her husband's hands, and some say on the wife's as well. (1982: 31)

16. Almost all of the twenty unmarried male students at the University of Zambia interviewed in 2002 said that their girlfriends cleaned them and

they cleaned their girlfriends. It is unclear whether they would continue to do this, once married.
17. Colson records the sentiment "Your wife is your mother" expressed by Tonga informants (1958: 140) and at local courts (1958: 205). Dover reports a similar popular saying among the Goba, "A good wife is like a second mother" (2001: 191).

CHAPTER 5

1. On the use of love potions to render men docile, see Epstein (1981: 351), Jules-Rosette (1981: 148), and Keller (1976).
2. From focus group discussions with women in Misisi township, Ndubani reports:

    > The women supported the view that most men in Misisi rarely used condoms unless they found that their sexual partner was coughing—coughing seemed to be a strong proxy for HIV in this community. They also pointed out that most men only used a condom during the initial sexual encounters with a new lover. They said that women could not persuade their husbands to use condoms except in situations where the woman "caught him red-handed with a prostitute." Then the husband would be obliged to use a condom with the wife. (2002: 37)

3. On the Bemba, see Richards (1969: 88):

    > In theory a woman cannot divorce her husband for adultery. Women laugh at the idea of a wife suing her husband on this ground, and women shrug their shoulders, and say that adultery is the way of men (*umusango wabo*). In fact both sexes are ready to admit that adultery is no ground for divorce. But at the same time Bemba women are also extremely jealous. They use magic to win and keep their husband's love exclusively and to inflict injury on rivals or co-wives.

    Colson records that among Plateau Tonga it was considered natural that a mature adult, either man or woman, would at some time be involved in adultery. She comments, "In former days, indeed, it seems to have been regarded as something bordering on the unnatural if a mature person died without being charged with adultery, *bulale*" (1958: 166). At the funeral steps were taken to correct the situation with a mock case brought against the deceased. Among other Tonga, men did not view a wife's adultery with such equanimity.
4. Abortion in Zambia is legal on medical and social grounds under the 1972 *Termination of Pregnancy Act*. However, Koster-Oyekan (1998) outlines why many women wanting an abortion do not have recourse to hospitals in the first instance.
5. The marriage later ended in divorce when Henry discovered that Pamela had started a relationship with another man.

6. Kitchen parties are all-women affairs at which household gifts are presented, alcohol is consumed, and advice to the bride-to-be is liberally given in a bawdy manner. Several husbands complained about the amount of money wives spent on kitchen party gifts and the indecorous behavior of some women at these parties. Hansen describes kitchen parties in Lusaka as a "loose version of initiation ceremonies" in which the bride-to-be has to demonstrate her skills at "dancing in bed" (1996: 134–135). She observes: "Given the male authoritarian atmosphere that characterizes sociality across all class levels in Zambia, it comes as no surprise that men blame kitchen parties as events where married women get drunk and engage in social evils, such as exposing unmarried women to offensive songs about sex and gossip about extra-marital relationships" (ibid.: 136).
7. Eating arrangements differed. In some households men ate separately. At the beginning of my stay in many homes, I was expected to eat separately with the male head of the household. If he was absent, I was required to eat alone. Women and children ate in the kitchen. During lengthy stays in some homes, however, occasionally almost the whole household—or as many as could fit around the table—would eat together.
8. Richards noted that control of food in rural Bemba households was considered a female skill at which older women were said to excel (1939: 88).
9. See Sobo (1995) on African-American women who, to preserve their own sense of self-worth, preferred denial to the acknowledgment that their partners' sexual activities put them at risk of HIV.
10. Other women might more readily seek divorce to protect themselves from an unreliable husband. For rural women increasingly choosing such an option in Malawi, see Smith and Watkins (2005).

Chapter 6

1. There has been extensive discussion of whether a distinctively "African sexuality" exists, as Caldwell and Caldwell (1987) and Caldwell et al. (1989) have proposed. See Le Blanc et al. (1991), Ahlberg (1994), Heald (1995), all of whom take the Caldwells to task for screening from view local moral understandings of sex. The Caldwells portray "traditional" African sexuality as one in which the conjugal bond is emotionally weak, women exchange sex with men for material goods, and money and sexual conduct is not subject to moral control. They contend that the spread of HIV/AIDS can be readily understood in a context in which little guilt is attached to sex and in which opportunities for sexual networking are increasing. The Caldwells defend themselves against anticipated accusations of racism, but the scope for such accusations is evident. (See Chirimuuta and Chirimuuta 1987 and Patton 1990.)

2. For such self-denigration of Zambian or "African" persons and things in 1990s Zambia, see Simpson (2003: 120) and Ferguson (1997) and (1999). The portrayal of Africans as lacking in self-control has a long history. For colonial portrayals, see Vaughan (1991: 284). For a notorious example from Northern Rhodesia, see Ritchie (1943).
3. Later cohorts of students made very similar evaluations (see Simpson 2003: 120).
4. Richards describes the shocked reaction of Bemba people: "White men and women eat and play together, formerly a mark of loose conduct among the Bemba. They may exchange endearments in public or dance in each other's arms—both shameful according to Native etiquette" (1969: 26). In recent years I have seen boyfriends and girlfriends holding hands and behaving in an openly affectionate manner (though they stop short of kissing) in the street and in public places in urban areas, especially in the capital Lusaka.
5. Darius's comment ironically, if unknowingly, echoes some elements of Caldwell et al.'s portrayal of "African sexuality": "[Sex] is a worldly activity like work or eating or drinking" (Caldwell et al. 1989: 203).
6. "Wet sex" was not disliked by *all* men in Zambia, or in the region more generally. See Taylor (1990).
7. See Simpson (2002) for *muti* used by boys and young men in rural Zambia. The term "gunpowder" is another example of the violent imagery that men (and at least some women) employed in discussing sexual intercourse.
8. Such intravaginal practices have been reported in eleven countries in sub-Saharan Africa. See van de Wijgert et al. who record that almost all their women respondents in Zimbabwe "reported that they themselves (89%) and their sexual partner(s) (94%) enjoyed sex very much after wiping" (2001: 138). See also Brown et al. (1993) on practices in central Zaire (now the Democratic Republic of Congo) that make the vagina "tight and dry" in preparation for penetration. They note that both men and women said this increased pleasure.
9. Richards records Bemba girls aged between twelve and fifteen meeting together in small groups to practice *ukukuna* (the enlargement of the labia by stretching) and comments upon their speaking earnestly about their duty to prepare for marriage in this way (1969: 16). Colson records labia enlargement among pre- and postpuberty girls, though she observes, "enlarged labia are said to give added sexual enjoyment to both men and women" (1958: 274). Parikh (2005) discusses a shift in some Ugandan women's understanding of this practice, from preparation to give men pleasure and to ease childbirth to a greater focus on women's sexual pleasure.
10. Chipata is the administrative center for Zambia's Eastern Province.
11. Ndubani reports that in all women focus group discussions in Misisi township, Lusaka, "a real man" was described as follows: "Sexually, he

must be a man who 'makes more rounds.' They said that, in bed, he should be *moto* (fire). A real man ejaculated proper semen, which they said, felt hot and made the woman weak soon after sex" (2002: 37).
12. Richards (1969) indicates that withdrawal was accepted practice in Bemba marriages following the birth of a child: "After the birth the father must refrain from normal sex intercourse with his wife until the child is weaned, although after some months, when the ceremony of the *ukupoko mwana* has been performed, *coitus interruptus* can be resumed. Any breaking of this taboo is considered as endangering the child's life and the father can be held liable for damages if it dies." (1969: 89) Data from the 2001–2002 Zambia Demographic and Health Survey estimate that withdrawal, described as a "traditional method," was currently practiced by 5% of currently married women, in contrast to 12% who used the pill (Central Statistical Office of Zambia 2003: xxii).
13. There was no suggestion that inserter, unlike the insertee, might retain his masculinity, as has been reported in Latin America. See Parker (1999) and Lancaster (1992). However, Moodie's account of South African mine marriages between older and younger men, who were seen as their wives, makes it clear that the "wife" was expected to remain passive and receptive while the "husband" ejaculated between the thighs. (1994: 127).
14. Here Promise hints that such behavior might well be associated with witchcraft.
15. I did not discuss oral and anal sex with students in my 1980s interviews. In the early 1980s students at St. Antony's were shocked by an expatriate woman teacher who spoke about oral sex in a biology lesson. They appeared genuinely amazed that human beings might engage in, and enjoy, oral sex.
16. See Mane and Aggleton (2000) for similar observations about "wasting semen" reported by women of their male sexual partners in Senegal. Dover (2001: 216) records Goba men's perceptions of semen as "a precious substance" in connection with some men's practice of cutting a hole in the top of the condom.
17. Homosexual acts are criminal offences in Zambia with possible sentences, on conviction, of more than ten years imprisonment.
18. A white homosexual character in a South African soap screened on Zambian television regularly provoked anger from television viewers. In one of the homes where I lived during fieldwork, there were repeated comments that he should be killed because of his homosexuality.
19. A story repeated many times over the years, of Lebanese men filming Zambian women having sex with dogs, was another indication of Lebanese men being portrayed as perverted. The circulation of these stories and their ready acceptance is perhaps an indication of a general feeling among Zambians of being exploited by, and consequent resentment toward, wealthy Lebanese who had successful business enterprises including stores and food outlets in urban areas.

20. It is difficult to exaggerate the value many Zambians place on fine clothes in the presentation of the self.
21. He did not appear to extend this suspicion to me.
22. Around Church Road in Lusaka there are a number of five-star hotels. On any night of the week, scantily dressed women could be seen adopting various poses, inviting men for sex. One of the hotels denied entrance to women unaccompanied by men. This was overruled by a successful challenge in court. (See Tamale 2001.)
23. Sampa uses the term "live" here to mean real, rather than, as elsewhere, sex without a condom.
24. Among the contraceptives that women took were *Norplant*, *Microgynon*, *Microrut*, and *Safe Plan*.
25. The definition of an immoral person was someone who was selfish. Ranked above all antisocial behavior, selfishness was the quintessential characteristic of witches who chose to "eat alone."

Chapter 7

1. Of his research in Northern Tanzania, Setel (1999: 201) notes: "It is worth emphasizing that having multiple partners is not a risk for HIV transmission *per se*." He argues, "The popular perceptions embedded in the presumption [that 'promiscuity' was somehow inherently risky], however, did not admit the possibility of meaningfully altering risk without altering numbers of partners" (ibid.: 212).
2. Elizabeth worked on short-term contracts; at the end of each she was paid a gratuity. Like many Zambians, her husband was following a course of home study from a U.K. correspondence organization and had to send regular remittances.
3. Attention to precedence was very important for many Zambians, as it had been for earlier generations. (See Richards 1969, 1982.) With the exception of Pentecostals, when discussing the doctrine of the Trinity, students explained to me that they understood that, though there were three persons in one God, Father, Son, and Holy Spirit, the Spirit was evidently less important as he was always mentioned last.
4. No student spoke of praying to ancestors for such help, as has been reported among female secondary school students in Tanzania (Stambach 1998).
5. See Colson (2004: 5) and Hinfelaar (1994: 6 note 7).
6. Smoking and drinking alcohol were singled out in Adventist teaching as sins against the body, the temple of the Spirit.
7. Some students suspected elderly villagers living near St. Antony's of using witchcraft to turn themselves into crocodiles in order to kill and eat children. During 2002 fieldwork in Northern Zambia, when I stayed in one home near a large river, my host family and neighbors sternly warned me about similar dangers. They insisted that I should not take walks alone along the riverbank.

8. This notion would later appear with rumors about AIDS sufferers deliberately infecting others so that they would not "die alone."
9. See Setel (1999: 240), Schoepf (1995), and Iliffe (2006: 80).
10. See Ogden (1996) on women, respect, and morality in postcolonial Kampala.
11. Liddell et al. (2005: 697) claim that to date no research has been undertaken in sub-Saharan Africa to discover whether indigenous attributions for AIDS actually influence people's decision-making in sexual situations. The contributors to a recent special issue of the *Journal of Religion in Africa* (2007) analyze the interaction between religion and AIDS in East Africa. Arguing for the intensification of involvement on the part of religious authorities in HIV/STD prevention at the local level, Lagarde et al. (2000) explore possible associations between religion and HIV prevention among Muslims and Christians in rural Senegal. They conclude that individuals who considered religion to be very important were not more likely to report intending to or actually having become faithful to protect themselves from AIDS. They highlight significant gender differences. While men who considered religion very important were less likely to feel at risk of getting HIV, women were less likely to report an intention to change to protect themselves from AIDS and yet were much more likely to feel at risk of getting HIV. Analyzing the 1998 Ghana Demographic Health Survey, Takyi (2003) concludes that while women's religious affiliation had a significant effect on knowledge about AIDS, it was not associated with changes in specific protective behavior, particularly the use of condoms. Agadjanian (2005) employs logistic regression to examine the effects of gender and of the interactions between gender and type of denomination in Mozambique—"mainline" (Catholic and Presbyterian) or "healing" (Assembly of God, Zionist, and Apostolic)—on male and female members' exposure to HIV/AIDS-related prevention messages, knowledge and perception of risks, and practices of prevention. He detects women's disadvantage on several measures of knowledge and prevention but notes that gender differences are less pronounced in "mainline" churches.
12. Hill et al.'s (2004) analysis of the 1996 Brazilian Demographic and Health Survey reveals that compared with members of evangelical religions, other men were significantly more likely to report having had an extramarital partner and unprotected extramarital sex in the last twelve months. They also note that region of residence was strongly correlated with extramarital sex.
13. Richards noted of Bemba sociality in the 1930s: "Bemba admire...the avoidance of quarrels, unpleasantness and 'scenes' which might disturb the delicate balance of village relations....They delight in circumlocutions...." (1982: 47).
14. Some readers might suggest that they phrased their discussions in this way because they were talking to their former teacher, whom they might assume would be critical of such activity. However, given our long-term

relationship, and what the men knew of me, I doubt that they perceived me simply as a judgmental observer for whom they needed to produce pious accounts.
15. While practicing Catholics had similar membership in what were called Small Christian Communities (*fitente*), only one former student in this group belonged to them.
16. See Montgomery et al. (2006) for an account of men's involvement in households affected by HIV/AIDS in rural KwaZulu Natal.

CHAPTER 8

1. This signaled a significant shift in Zambian ways of grieving. Formerly, it would have been unthinkable not to make every effort to attend the funeral of all family members, friends, and work colleagues, no matter how distant the burial or what expense might be involved.
2. I asked all former students in the study whether they had had a test, though I stressed that I was not seeking to know the result. Their reluctance to be tested was not atypical. See Fylkesnes et al. (1999).
3. This scaling up of the ARV treatment program has been heralded as one of the most successful in the world (*New York Times*, 13 August 2006).
4. There are echoes of earlier attitudes toward women without a male partner in urban areas throughout the region. See White (1990).
5. See Baggaley et al. (1996) on HIV counselors in Lusaka.
6. The term "the animal in man" was a familiar phrase from Kaunda's philosophy of Christian Humanism.
7. See Barnett and Whiteside (2002: 227ff) for the impact of HIV/AIDS on rural areas in sub-Saharan Africa.
8. The papal encyclical *Evangelium Vitae* (The Gospel of Life) spoke of "the moral unlawfulness of contraception" and the "negative values inherent in the 'contraceptive mentality'" (1995: 23). However, there were dissenting voices among some Catholic missionaries working in AIDS education, prevention, and care in Zambia.
9. "Social life" is a commonly used euphemism in Zambia for sexual activity.
10. His wife had, without his knowledge, asked me to speak to him about the risk of contracting and transmitting the HIV virus to her.
11. The American President's Emergency Plan for AIDS Relief (PEPFAR) was launched in 2003. Among the aims, in the planned investment of U.S. $15 billion, was the promotion of abstinence.
12. This contrasts strikingly with, for example, rural Bemba marriage in the first part of the twentieth century. Richards observed: "Bemba men and women can leave their partners fairly easily, for there are no complicated marriage payments to be returned" (1982: 156).

Chapter 9

1. Connell observes, "Bodily experience is often central in memories of our own lives, and thus in our understanding of who and what we are" (1995: 53) and "the bodily sense of masculinity is central to the social process" (ibid.: 123).
2. This ritual symbolic code in the initiation of boys and girls is reported elsewhere in the region. Kaspin (1999) draws attention to the Chewa puberty rites of Nyau in Malawi where boys are taught to become predators who hunt and eat all kinds of meat and girls learn that they are the game that men hunt.
3. See Kaufman (1998: 8) on male power and emotional isolation. Connell (2000: 173) and Barker (2005) make similar observations.
4. While, for young people in formal education, the school may offer a forum where issues of gender and power may be usefully debated, the school may be marked with local gendered regimes of discipline and power that make it an unpromising space for dialogue. Deacon et al. (1999) describe the role of local disciplinary mechanisms in South African schools. Students also generate their own gender regimes that may differ significantly from those promoted by the school administration. (See Simpson 2003: 128–134, for an account of such a process at St. Antony's.) At times, spaces beyond the classroom may be more conducive to explorations of gender and power. However, in South Africa *Dramaide* (an acronym for Drama in AIDS education) is a successful intervention that has been documented and analyzed (Dalrymple 1996; Dalrymple and Jaffe 1996). Tapping into local expressions of oral tradition, dance, and song, *Dramaide* uses a mix of performance theatre-in-education, forum theatre, and arts workshop. A further development, which employs forum theatre techniques (see Boal 1995), is the Act-Alive program with its broader workshops for Brazilian teenagers.
5. See Holland et al. (1998: 191) for the consequences of this division for vulnerability to sexual risk among young women and men in Britain.
6. The pilot project in Zambia was partly financed by Save the Children (Sweden and South Africa). It was conducted in a high school (grades seven to twelve), three basic schools (grades one to nine), and three teacher training colleges in 2002. The Zambian Ministry of Education chose the schools and colleges. Sessions were also conducted with in-service teachers and Education Ministry personnel. For discussion and analysis of the project, see Simpson and Heap (2002) and Heap and Simpson (2004, 2005), from which some extracts have been taken.
7. See also Leclerc-Madlala (2002); Paiva (2000); Parker, Barbosa, and Aggleton (2000).
8. For examples of such work in Africa, see Schoepf (1993); Obbo (1995); Seidel and Coleman (1999). Process drama that is carefully documented may produce findings that critique aspects of existing HIV/AIDS campaigns and suggest alternative approaches.

9. See Weeks on British students who temporarily took up an anti-homophobic stance: "[T]hey momentarily inhabited this alternative world-view, and thus created, for themselves, the possibility of inhabiting it again in the future" (1999: 39).
10. The majority of the pupils who participated at this school were in the seventeen to nineteen age group. I use the terminology "boy" and "girl," although the majority of pupils were in their late teens, not as it might be in school settings to insist on the puerility of the pupils. Rather it is used because this is the manner with which pupils identified themselves and their classmates, a reflection of their acknowledgment that, despite their age, they continued to be dependants of their parents and other guardians.
11. See Sabo and Gordon (1995: 16); Setel (1999: 245).
12. See Barnett (1999) for the use of this term to signal the long-term consequences of HIV/AIDS.

References

Adams, Vincanne and Stacy Leigh Pigg. ed. 2005. *Sex in Development: Science, Sexuality, and Morality in Global Perspective*. Durham and London: Duke University Press.

Agadjanian, V. 2005. "Gender, Religious Involvement, and HIV/AIDS Prevention in Mozambique." *Social Science and Medicine* 61: 1529–1539.

Ahlberg, Beth, M. 1994. "Is There a Distinct African Sexuality? A Critical Response to Caldwell et al." *Africa* 64: 220–242.

Ahlberg, Beth. M., Eila Jylkas, and Ingela Krantz. 2001. "Gendered Construction of Sexual Risks: Implications for Safer Sex among Young People in Kenya and Sweden." *Reproductive Health Matters* 9 (17): 26–36.

Akeroyd, Anne. V. 1997. "Sociocultural Aspects of AIDS in Africa: Occupational and Gender Issues." In *AIDS in Africa and the Caribbean*, ed. George C. Bond, John Kreniske, Ida Susser, and Joan Vincent. 11–32. Boulder: Westview Press.

Ankrah, E. Maxine. 1991. "AIDS and the Social Side of Health." *Social Science and Medicine* 32 (9): 967–980.

Auslander, Mark. 1993. "'Open the Wombs': The Symbolic Politics of Modern Ngoni Witchfinding." In *Modernity and Its Malcontents: Ritual and Power in Postcolonial Africa*, ed. Jean and John Comaroff. 167–192. Chicago: University of Chicago Press.

Baggaley, R., J. Sulwe, M. Kelly, M. Macmillan Ndovi, and P. Godfrey-Faussett. 1996. "HIV Counsellors' Knowledge, Attitudes and Vulnerabilities to HIV in Lusaka, Zambia, 1994." *AIDS Care* 8 (2): 155–166.

Barker, Gary, T. 2005. *Dying to Be Men: Youth, Masculinity and Social Exclusion*. London and New York: Routledge.

Barnett, Tony. 1999. "HIV/AIDS: Long Wave Event, Short Wave Event: Identity, Gender, Agriculture and Policy in Uganda and Elsewhere". Paper presented at American Anthropological Association Annual Meeting in Chicago, 17–20 November 1999.

Barnett, Tony and Alan Whiteside. 2002. *AIDS in the Twenty-First Century: Disease and Globalisation*. Hampshire: Palgrave-MacMillan.

Bawa Yamba, C. 1997. "Cosmologies in Turmoil: Witchfinding and AIDS in Chiawa, Zambia." *Africa* 67 (2): 200–223.

References

Bayley, Anne C. 1984. "Aggressive Kaposi's Sarcoma in Zambia." *The Lancet* i: 1318–1320.

———. 1996. *One New Humanity: Challenge of AIDS*. London: SPCK.

Bayley, A. C., R. G. Downing, R. Cheingsong-Popov, R. S. Tedder, A. G. Dalgleish, and R. A. Weiss. 1985. "HTLV-III Serology Distinguishes Atypical and Endemic Kaposi's Sarcoma in Africa." *The Lancet* i: 360.

Baylies, Carolyn and Janet Bujra, with the Gender and AIDS Group. 2000. *AIDS, Sexuality and Gender in Africa: Collective Strategies and Struggles in Tanzania and Zambia*. London and New York: Routledge.

Becker, Felicitas and P. Wenzel Geissler. 2007. "Searching for Pathways in a Landscape of Death: Religion and AIDS in East Africa." *Journal of Religion in Africa* 37: 1–15.

Berger, Maurice, Brian Wallis, and Simon Watson, eds. 1995. *Constructing Masculinity*. New York and London: Routledge.

Boal, Augusto. 1996. "Politics, Education and Change." In *Drama, Culture and Empowerment*, ed. J. O'Toole and K. Donelan. 47–52. Brisbane: IDEA Publications.

Bolton, Ralph. 1992. "Mapping Terra Incognita: Sex Research for AIDS Prevention—an Urgent Agenda for the 1990s." In *The Time of AIDS: Social Analysis, Theory and Method*, ed. Gilbert Herdt and Shirley Lindenbaum. 124–158. London: Sage Publications.

———. 1995. "Rethinking Anthropology: The Study of AIDS." In *Culture and Sexual Risk*, ed. Han Ten Brummelhuis and Gilbert Herdt. New York and Amsterdam: Gordon and Breach.

Bond, V. A. and P. Dover. 1997. "Men, Women and the Trouble with Condoms: Problems Associated with Condom Use by Migrant Workers in Rural Zambia." *Health Transition Review* 7 (Supplement): 377–391.

Bowell, Pamela and Brian Heap. 2001. *Planning Process Drama*. London: David Fulton Publishers.

Brown, Judith. E., Okako Bibi Ayowa, and Richard C. Brown. 1993. "Dry and Tight: Sexual Practices and Potential AIDS Risk in Zaire." *Social Science and Medicine* 37 (8): 989–994.

Bruner, Jerome. 1986. *Actual Minds, Possible Worlds*. Cambridge, MA: Harvard University Press.

Bujra, Janet. 2000. "Risk and Trust: Unsafe Sex, Gender and AIDS in Tanzania." In *Risk Revisited*, ed. Pat Caplan. 59–84. London: Pluto Press.

Burke, Timothy. 1996. *Lifebuoy Men, Lux Women: Commodification, Consumption and Cleanliness in Modern Zimbabwe*. Durham, N.C. and London: Duke University Press.

Butler, Judith. 1990. *Gender Trouble*. New York and London: Routledge.

———. 1993. *Bodies That Matter: On the Discursive Limits of Sex*. New York and London: Routledge.

Buvé, A., M. Caraël, R. J. Hayes, B. Auvert, B. Ferry, N. J. Robinson, S. Anagonou, L. Kanhonou, M. Laourou, S. Abega, E. Akam, L. Zekeng, J. Chege, M. Kahindo, N. Rutenberg, F. Kaona, R. Musonda, T. Sukwa, L. Morison, H. A. Weiss, and M. Laga, for the Study Group on Heterogeneity of HIV Epidemics in African Cities. 2001. "Multicentre Study on Factors Determining Differences in Rate of Spread of HIV in Sub-Saharan Africa: Methods and Prevalence of HIV Infection." *AIDS* 15 (4): S5–S14.

Caldwell, J. C. and P. Caldwell. 1987. "The Cultural Context of High Fertility in Sub-Saharan Africa." *Population and Development Review* 13: 409–437.

Caldwell, J. C., P. Caldwell, and P. Quiggin. 1989. "The Social Context of AIDS in Sub-Saharan Africa." *Population and Development Review* 15: 185–234.

Campbell, Carole A. 1995. "Male Gender Roles and Sexuality: Implications for Women's AIDS Risk and Prevention." *Social Science and Medicine* 41 (2): 197–210.

Campbell, Catherine. 1992. "Learning to Kill? Masculinity, the Family and Violence in Natal." *Journal of Southern African Studies* 18 (3): 614–628.

Caplan, Pat. 1997. *African Voices, African Lives: Personal Narratives from a Swahili Village*. London and New York: Routledge.

Central Statistical Office of Zambia. 2003. *Zambia Demographic and Health Survey (2001–2002)*. http://www.zamstats.gov.zm.

Chapman, Rowena and Jonathan Rutherford. 1988. *Male Order: Unwrapping Masculinity*. London: Lawrence and Wishart.

Chirimuuta, Richard C. and Rosalind J. Chirimuuta. 1987. *AIDS, Africa and Racisms*. Bretby: R. C. Chirimuuta.

Clatts, Michael C. 1994. "All the Kings Horses and All the King's Men: Some Personal Reflections on Ten Years of AIDS Ethnography." *Human Organization* 53 (1): 93–95.

Cohen, Anthony 1996. "Against the Motion: Anthropology Is a Generalising Science or It Is Nothing." In *Key Debates in Anthropology*, ed. Tim Ingold. 26–30. London: Routledge.

Colson, Elizabeth. 1958. *Marriage and the Family among the Plateau Tonga*. Manchester: Manchester University Press.

———. 2000. "The Father as Witch." *Africa* 70 (3): 333–358.

———. 2004. "*Leza* into God—God into *Leza*." In *Religion and Education in Zambia*, ed. Brendan Carmody. 1–7. Ndola, Zambia: Mission Press.

Connell, Robert. 1983. *Which Way Is Up? Essays on Class, Sex and Culture*. Sydney: Allen and Unwin.

———. 1995. *Masculinities*. Cambridge: Polity Press.

———. 2000. *The Men and the Boys*. London: Polity Press.

Dählback, Elisabeth, Patrick Makele, Phillimon Ndubani, Bawa Yamba, Staffan Bergström, and Anna-Berit Ransjö-Arvidson. 2003. "'I Am Happy that God Made Me a Boy': Zambian Adolescent Boys' Perceptions about Growing into Manhood." *African Journal of Reproductive Health* 7 (1): 49–62.

Dalrymple, L. 1996. "In the Fight against AIDS, Theatre Empowers Children to Educate Their Own Communities." In *Drama, Culture and Empowerment*, ed. J. O'Toole and K. Donelan. 33–35. Brisbane: IDEA Publications.

Dalrymple, L. and A. Jaffe. 1996. "Dramaide, A Project in Schools in Kwazulu-Natal, South Africa." In *Aids Education Interventions in Multi-Cultural Societies*, ed. I. I. Schenker, G. Saber-Friedman, and F. S. Sy. 119–123. New York and London: Plenum Press.

Deacon, R., R. Morrell, and J. Prinslo. 1999. "Discipline and Homophobia in South African Schools: The Limits of Legislated Transformation." In *A Dangerous Knowing: Sexuality, Pedagogy and Popular Culture*, ed. Debbie Epstein and James T. Sears. 164–175. London: Continuum.

de Bruyn, M. 1992. "Women and AIDS in Developing Countries." *Social Science and Medicine* 34 (2): 249–262.

Delius, Peter and Clive Glaser. 2002. "Sexual Socialisation in South Africa: A Historical Perspective." *African Studies* 61 (1): 27–54.

Dillon-Malone, Clive. 2004: "Is HIV/AIDS a Punishment from God?" *Jesuit Centre for Theological Reflection Bulletin* 59 (1): 9–11.

DiPiero, Thomas. 2002. *White Men Aren't*. Durham and London: Duke University Press.

Douglas, Mary. 1966. *Purity and Danger: An Analysis of Conceptions of Pollution and Taboo*. London: Routledge and Kegan Paul.

Dover, Paul. 2001. *Man of Power*. Unpublished Ph.D. thesis, Department of Cultural Anthropology and Ethnology, Uppsala University, Sweden.

———. 2005. "Gender and Embodiment: Expectations of Manliness in a Zambian Village." In *African Masculinities: Men in Africa from the Late Nineteenth Century to the Present*, ed. Lahoucine Ouzgane and Robert Morrell. 173–187. Scottsville, South Africa: University of KwaZulu-Natal Press.

Dowsett, Gary. 1999. "The Indeterminate Macro-Social: New Traps for Old Players in HIV/AIDS Social Research." *Culture, Health and Sexuality* 1 (1): 95–102.

Doyal, Leslie, Sara Paparini, and Jane Anderson. 2008. "'Elvis Died and I Was Born': Black African Men Negotiating Same-Sex Desire in London." *Sexualities* 11 (1/2): 171–192.

Epstein, Arnold L. 1981. *Urbanisation and Kinship: The Domestic Domain on the Copperbelt of Zambia, 1950–1956*. London and New York: New Academic Press.

———. 1992. *Scenes from African Urban Life: Collected Copperbelt Papers*. Edinburgh: Edinburgh University Press.

Fanon, Frantz. 1967. *Black Skin, White Masks*. Translated by Charles Lam Markmann. New York: Grove.

Farmer, Paul. 1997. "AIDS and Anthropologists: Ten Years Later." *Medical Anthropology Quarterly* 11 (4): 516–525.

Feldman, Douglas, Peggy O'Hara, K. S. Baboo, Ndashi Chitalu, and Lu Ying. 1997. "HIV Prevention among Zambian Adolescents: Developing a Value Utilization/Norm Change Model." *Social Science and Medicine* 44 (4): 4455–4468.

Ferguson, James. 1997. "The Country and the City on the Copperbelt." In *Culture, Power and Place: Ethnography at the End of an Era*,

ed. Akhil Gupta and James Ferguson. 137–154. Durham: Duke University Press.
———. 1999. *Expectations of Modernity*. Berkeley: University of California Press.
Fetters, Tamara, Evans Mupela, and Naomi Rutenberg. 1997. *"Don't Trust Your Girlfriend or You're Gonna Die Like a Chicken": A Participatory Assessment of Adolescent Sexual Risk and Reproductive Health in a High Risk Environment*. CARE Zambia Operations Research (mimeo).
Flood, Michael. 2003. "Lust, Trust and Latex: Why Young Heterosexual Men Do not Use Condoms." *Culture, Health and Sexuality* 5 (4): 353–369.
Foreman, Martin. 1999. *AIDS and Men, Taking Risks or Taking Responsibility?* London: Panos/Zed.
Fortes, Meyer. 1974. "The First Born." *Journal of Child Psychology, Psychiatry and Allied Disciplines* 15: 81–104.
Foucault, M. 1979. *The History of Sexuality Volume One: An Introduction*. Translated by R. Hurley. London: Allen Lane.
Frankenberg, Ronald. 1995. "Learning from AIDS: The Future of Anthropology." In *The Future of Anthropology: Its Relevance to the Contemporary World*, ed. A. Ahmed and C. Shore. 110–133. London: Athlone Press.
Freire, Paolo. 1983. *Education for Critical Consciousness*. New York: Seabury Press and Continuum Press.
Fylkesnes, K., A. Haworth, C. Rosenvärd, and P. M. Kwapa. 1999. "HIV Counselling and Testing: Overemphasing High Acceptance Rates a Threat to Confidentiality and the Right to Know." *AIDS* 13 (17): 2469–2427.
Garner, Robert. C. 2000. "Safe Sects? Dynamic Religion and AIDS in South Africa." *Journal of Modern African Studies* 38 (1): 41–69.
Geschiere, Peter and Cyprian Fisiy. 1994. "Domesticating Personal Violence: Witchcraft, Courts and Confessions in Cameroon." *Africa* 64 (3): 323–341.
Goffman, Erving. 1959. *The Presentation of Self in Everyday Life*. Garden City, NY: Doubleday Anchor.
———. 1963. *Stigma: Notes on the Management of Spoiled Identity*. New York: Simon and Schuster Inc.
———. 1974. *Frame Analysis: An Essay on the Organization of Experience*. Cambridge, MA: Harvard University Press.
Green, Gill and Elisa J. Sobo. 2000. *The Endangered Self: Managing the Social Risks of HIV*. London and New York: Routledge.
Gutmann, Matthew. C. 1997. "Trafficking in Men: The Anthropology of Masculinity." *Annual Review of Anthropology* 26: 385–409.
Hall, Stuart. 1996. "Introduction: Who Needs Identity?" In *Questions of Cultural Identity*, ed. Stuart Hall and Paul Du Gay. 1–17. London: Sage.
Hansen, Karen. 1996. *Keeping House in Lusaka*. New York: Columbia University Press.

Heald, Suzette. 1995. "The Power of Sex: Some Reflections on the Caldwell's 'African Sexuality' Thesis." *Africa* 65 (4): 489–505.
———. 1999. *Manhood and Morality: Sex, Violence and Ritual in Gisu Society*. London: Routledge.
———. 2002. "It's Never as Easy as ABC: Understandings of AIDS in Botswana." *African Journal of AIDS Research* 1: 1–10.
Heap, Brian and Anthony Simpson. 2004. " 'When You Have AIDS People Laugh at You': A Process Drama Approach to Stigma with Pupils in Zambia." *Caribbean Quarterly* 50 (1): 83–98.
———. 2005 "A Lesson for the Living: Promoting HIV/AIDS Competence among Young Zambians." *Youth Theatre Journal* 19: 89–101.
Heathcote, Dorothy. 1984. *Collected Writings on Education and Drama*. Evanston, IL: Northwestern University Press.
Heise, L., A. Raikes, C. Watts, and A. Zwi. 1994. "Violence against women: A Neglected Public Health Issue in Less Developed Countries." *Social Science and Medicine* 39 (9): 1165–1179.
Herdt, Gilbert. 1997. "Sexual Cultures and Population Movement: Implications for AIDS/STDs." In *Sexual Cultures and Migration in the Era of AIDS: Anthropological and Demographic Perspectives*, ed. Gilbert Herdt. 3–22. Oxford: Clarendon Press.
Herzfeld, Michael. 1985. *The Poetics of Manhood: Contest and Identity in a Cretan Mountain Village*. Princeton: Princeton University Press.
Heward, Catherine. 1988. *Making a Man of Him: Parents and Their Sons' Education at an English Public School, 1929–1950*. London: Routledge.
Hill, A. E., J. Cleland, and M. M. Ali. 2004. "Religious Affiliation and Extramarital Sex among Men in Brazil." *International Family Planning Perspectives* 30 (1): 20–26.
Hinfelaar, Hugo F. 1994. *Bemba-Speaking Women in Zambia in a Century of Religious Change*. Leiden: Brill.
Hira, S. K., U. Mangrola, C. Mwale, C. Chintu, G. Tembo, W. E. Brady, and P. L. Perine. 1990. "Apparent Vertical Transmission of Human Immunodeficiency Virus Type 1 by Breast-Feeding in Zambia." *Clinical and Laboratory Observations* 117: 421–424.
Holland, Janet, Caroline Ramazanoglu, Sue Sharpe, and Rachel Thomson. 1998. *The Male in the Head: Young People, Sexuality and Power*. London: The Tufnell Press.
Hunter, Mark. 2002. "The Materiality of Everyday Sex: Thinking beyond 'Prostitution.' " *African Studies* 61 (1): 99–120.
Iliffe, John. 2006. *The African AIDS Epidemic: A History*. Oxford: James Currey.
Jacobson-Widding, Anita. 2000. *Chapungu: The Bird That Never Drops a Feather*. Uppsala: Uppsala University Library.
Jeater, Diana. 1993. *Marriage, Perversion and Power: The Construction of Moral Discourse in Southern Rhodesia 1894–1930*. Oxford: Clarendon.
Jules-Rosette, Benetta. 1981. *Symbols of Change, Urban Transition in a Zambian Community*. Norwood, NJ: Ablex Publishing Corporation.

REFERENCES

Kalipenta, J. and C. Chalowandya. 1995. *Southern Province Peer Education Programme, Groundwork Report, Pilot Study Areas: Mazabuka and Monze* (mimeo).
Kambou, Sarah Degnan, Meera Kaul Shah, and Gladys Nkhama. 1998. "For a Pencil: Sex and Adolescence in Peri-Urban Lusaka." In *The Myth of Community: Gender Issues in Participatory Development*, ed. Irene Guijit and Meera Kaul Shaw. London: Intermediate Technology Publications.
Kappeler, Susanne. 1986. *The Pornography of Representation*. Oxford: Polity Press.
Kaspin, Deborah. 1999. "The Lion at the Waterhole." In *Those Who Play with Fire: Gender, Fertility and Transformation in East and Southern Africa*, ed. Henrietta Moore, Todd Sanders, and Bwire Kaare. 41–82. London: Athlone Press.
Kaufman, Michael. 1998. "The Construction of Masculinity and the Triad of Men's Violence." In *Men's Lives*, ed. Michael S. Kimmel and M. A. Messner. Boston, MA and London: Allyn and Bacon.
Kaufman, Carol E. and Stavros E. Stavrou. 2004. "'Bus Fare Please': The Economics of Sex and Gifts among Young People in Urban South Africa." *Culture, Health and Sexuality* 6 (5): 377–391.
Keller, Bonnie. 1976. "Marriage and Medicine: Women's Search for Love and Luck." *African Social Research* 26: 489–505.
Kelly, Michael. 2000. "Standing Education on Its Head: Aspects of Schooling in a World with HIV/AIDS." *Current Issues in Contemporary Education* (CICE) 3 (1). New York Teachers' College, Columbia. www.tc.columbia.edu/cice.
Kimmel, Michael, ed. 1988. *Changing Men: New Directions in Research on Men and Masculinity*. Newbury Park, CA: Sage.
Kleinman, Arthur, Veena Das, and Margaret Lock, eds. 1997. *Social Suffering*. Berkeley: University of California Press.
Koster-Oyekan, Winny. 1998. "Why Resort to Illegal Abortion in Zambia? Findings of a Community-Based Study in Western Province." *Social Science and Medicine* 46 (10): 1303–1312.
Lagarde, E., C. Enel, K. Seck, A. Gueye-Ndiaye, J-P. Piau, G. Pison, V. Delaunay, I. Ndoye, and S. Mboup for the MECORA group. 2000. "Religion and Protective Behaviours towards AIDS in Rural Senegal." *AIDS* 14: 2027–2033.
Lancaster, Roger N. 1992. *Life Is Hard: Machismo, Danger and the Intimacy of Power in Nicaragua*. Berkeley: University of California Press.
Laqueur, Thomas. 2003. *Solitary Sex: A Cultural History of Masturbation*. New York and London: Zone; MIT.
Last, Murray. 2000. "Children and the Experience of Violence: Contrasting Cultures of Punishment in Northern Nigeria." *Africa* 70 (3): 359–393.
Laumann, Edward and John Gagnon. 1995. "A Sociological Perspective on Sexual Action." In *Conceiving Sexuality: Approaches to Sex Research in a Postmodern World*, ed. Richard Parker and John Gagnon. 183–214. New York: Routledge.

Le Blanc, Marie-Nathalie, Deirdre Meintel, and Victor Piche. 1991. "The African Sexual System: Comment on Caldwell et al." *Population and Development Review* 17 (3): 497–505.

Leclerc-Madlala, Susanne. 2002. "Youth, HIV/AIDS and the Importance of Sexual Culture and Context." *Social Dynamics* 28 (1): 20–40.

Liddell, C., L. Barrett, and M. Bydawell. 2005. "Indigenous Representations of Illness and AIDS in Sub-Saharan Africa." *Social Science and Medicine* 60: 691–700.

Lonsdale, John. 2007. "Conclusion." *Journal of Religion in Africa* 37: 145–149.

Lupton, Deborah. 1995. *The Imperative of Health: Public Health and the Regulated Body.* London: Sage.

Mair, Lucy. 1953. *Survey of African Marriage and Family Life.* London: Oxford University Press for the International African Institute.

Mane, Purnima and Peter Aggleton. 2000. "Cross-National Perspectives on Gender and Power." In *Framing the Sexual Subject: The Politics of Gender, Sexuality and Power*, ed. Richard Parker, Regina M. Barbosa, and Peter Aggleton. 104–116. Berkeley: University of California Press.

———. 2001. "Gender and HIV/AIDS: What Do Men Have to Do with It?" *Current Sociology* 49 (6): 23–37.

Manuel, Sandra. 2005. "Obstacles to Condom Use among Secondary School Students in Maputo City, Mozambique." *Culture, Health and Sexuality* 7 (3): 293–302.

Marks, Shula. 1989. "The Context of Personal Narrative: Reflections on 'Not Either an Experimental Doll.'" In *Interpreting Women's Lives: Feminist Theory and Personal Narratives*, ed. Personal Narratives Group. 39–57. Bloomington: Indiana University Press.

Mbilinyi, Marjorie. 1989. "'I'd Have Been a Man': Politics and the Labour Process in Producing Personal Narratives." In *Interpreting Women's Lives: Feminist Theory and Personal Narratives*, ed. Personal Narratives Group. 204–225. Bloomington: Indiana University Press.

Meigs, Anna. 1990. "Multiple Gender Ideologies and Statuses." In *Beyond the Second Sex: New Directions in the Anthropology of Gender*, ed. Peggy Reeves Sanday and Ruth Gallagher Goodenough. 101–112. Philadelphia: University of Pennsylvania Press.

Miescher, Stephan F. 2005. *Making Men in Ghana.* Bloomington and Indianapolis: Indiana University Press.

Mogensen, H. O. 1997. "The Narrative of AIDS among the Tonga of Zambia." *Social Science and Medicine* 44 (4): 431–439.

Montgomery, C. M., V. Hoosegood, J. Buisza, and I. M. Timaeus. 2006. "Men's Involvement in the South African Family: Engendering Change in the AIDS Era." *Social Science and Medicine* 62: 2411–2419.

Moodie, Dunbar T. with Vivienne Ndatshe. 1994. *Going for Gold: Men, Mines and Migration.* Berkeley: University of California Press.

Moore, Henrietta and Megan Vaughan. 1994. *Cutting Down Trees: Gender, Nutrition and Agricultural Change in the Northern Province of Zambia, 1890–1990.* Portsmouth, NH and Heinemann/London: James Currey.

Morrell, Robert and Sandra Swart. 2005. "Men in the Third World: Postcolonial Perspectives on Masculinity." In *Handbook of Studies on Men and Masculinities*, ed. Michael S. Kimmel, Jeff Hearn, and R. W. Connell. 90–113. Thousand Oaks: Sage Publications.

Mufune, Pempelani, Kwaku Osei-Hwedie, and Lengwe-Katembula Mwansa. 1993. "Attitudes toward Risky Sexual Behavior and Reactions to People Infected with HIV among Zambian Students." *International Family Planning Perspectives* 19: 25–30.

Muvandi, I., P. Dover, and A. Ilinigumugabo. n.d. *Heads, Tails or Equality?: Men, Women and Reproductive Health in Zambia.* Online. Available at: www.popline.org/docs/1501/192653.

Mwanakatwe, John M. 1968. *The Growth of Education in Zambia since Independence.* Oxford: Oxford University Press.

Ndubani, Phillimon. 2002. *Young Men's Sexuality and Sexually Transmitted Infections in Zambia.* Stockholm: Karolinska University Press.

Niehaus, Isaak. 2000. "Towards a Dubious Liberation: Masculinity, Sexuality and Power in South African Lowveld Schools, 1953–1999." *Journal of Southern African Studies* 26 (3): 387–407.

Obbo, Caroline. 1993. "HIV Transmission: Men Are the Solution." *Population and Environment* 14 (3): 211–243.

———. 1995. "Gender, Age and Class: Discourses on HIV Transmission and Control in Uganda". In *Culture and Sexual Risk*, ed. H. ten Brummelhuis and Gilbert Herdt. New York and Amsterdam: Gordon and Breach.

Ogden, Jessica A. 1996. "'Producing' Respect: The 'Proper Woman' in Postcolonial Kampala." In *Postcolonial Identities in Africa*, ed. Richard Werbner and Terence Ranger. 165–192. London: Zed Press.

Okely, Judith. 1996. "Against the Motion: Anthropology Is a Generalising Science or It Is Nothing." In *Key Debates in Anthropology*, ed. Tim Ingold. 36–40. London: Routledge.

Paiva, V. 2000. "Gendered Scripts and the Sexual Scene: Promoting Sexual Subjects among Brazilian Teenagers." In *Framing the Sexual Subject: The Politics of Gender, Sexuality and Power*, ed. Richard Parker, Regina Barbosa, and Peter Aggleton. 216–239. Berkeley: University of California Press.

Parikh, Shanti A. 2005. "From Auntie to Disco: The Bifurcation of Risk and Pleasure in Sex Education in Uganda." In *Sex in Development: Science, Sexuality, and Morality in Global Perspective*, ed. Vincanne Adams and Stacy Leigh Pigg. 125–158. Durham and London: Duke University Press.

Parker, Richard G. 1992. "Sexual Diversity, Cultural Analysis and AIDS Education in Brazil." In *The Time of AIDS: Social Analysis, Theory and*

Method, ed. Gilbert Herdt and Shirley Lindenbaum. 225–242. London: Sage Publications.

Parker, Richard G. 1999. *Beneath the Equator: Cultures of Desire, Male Homosexuality and Emerging Gay Communities in Brazil*. London and New York: Routledge.

———. 2000. "Administering the Epidemic: HIV/AIDS Policy, Models of Development, and International Health." In *Global Health Policy, Local Realities*, ed. L. M. Whiteford and L. Manderson. 39–55. London: Lynne Rienner.

———. 2001. "Sexuality, Culture and Power in HIV/AIDS Research." *Annual Review of Anthropology* 30: 163–179.

Parker, Richard, Regina Barbosa, and Peter Aggleton, ed. 2000. *Framing the Sexual Subject: The Politics of Gender, Sexuality and Power*. Berkeley: University of California Press.

Pattman, Rob. 2001. " 'The Beer Drinkers Say I Had a Nice Prostitute but the Church Goers Talk about Things Spiritual'—Learning to Be Men at a Teachers' College in Zimbabwe." In *Changing Men in Southern Africa*, ed. Robert Morrell. 225–238. London: Zed Press Ltd/Pietermaritzburg: University of Natal Press.

Pattman, Rob and Fatuma Chege. 2003. " 'Dear Diary I Saw an Angel, She Looked Like Heaven on Earth': Sex Talk and Sex Education." *African Journal of AIDS Research* 2 (2): 99–108.

Patton, Cindy. 1990. *Inventing African AIDS*. New York and London: Routledge.

Pigg, Stacy Leigh and Vincanne Adams. 2005. "Introduction: The Moral Object of Sex." In *Sex in Development: Science, Sexuality, and Morality in Global Perspective*, ed. Vincanne Adams and Stacy Leigh Pigg. 1–38. Durham and London: Duke University Press.

Plummer, Ken. [1995] 1997. *Telling Sexual Stories: Power, Change and Social Worlds*. London and New York: Routledge.

———. 2005. "Male Sexualities." In *Handbook of Studies on Men and Masculinities*, ed. Michael S. Kimmel, Jeff Hearn, and R. W. Connell. 178–195. Thousand Oaks: Sage Publications.

Powdermaker, Hortense. 1962. *Coppertown: Changing Africa, the Human Situation on the Rhodesian Copperbelt*. New York: Harper and Row.

Rabinow, Paul. 1977. *Reflections on Fieldwork in Morocco*. Berkeley: University of California Press.

Ranger, Terence. 1992. "Plagues of Beasts and Men: Prophetic Responses to Epidemic in Eastern and Southern Africa." In *Epidemics and Ideas: Essays on the Historical Perception of Pestilence*, ed. Terence Ranger and Paul Slack. 241–268. Cambridge: Cambridge University Press.

Rasing, Thera. 1995. *Passing on the Rites of Passage*. Amsterdam: Avebury Press for the African Studies Centre, Leiden.

———. 2001. *The Bush Burnt, the Stones Remain: Female Initiation Rites in Urban Zambia*. Hamburg/Leiden: Lit Verlag/ASC.

REFERENCES

———. 2004. "HIV/AIDS and Sex Education among the Youth in Zambia: Towards Behavioural Change." Available at: www.hivaidsclearinghouse. unesco.org.

Reid, Elizabeth. 1997a. "Placing Women at the Center of Analysis." In *AIDS in Africa and the Caribbean*, ed. George C. Bond, John Kreniske, Ida Susser, and Joan Vincent. 159–164. Boulder: Westview Press.

———. 1997b. "HIV Prevention and Development in Multicultural Contexts." In *AIDS Education Interventions in Multi-Cultural Societies*, ed. I. I. Schenker, G. Saber-Friedman, and F. S. Sy. New York and London: Plenum Press.

Reynaud, E. 1981. *Holy Virility: The Social Construction of Masculinity*. London: Pluto.

Reynolds-Whyte, Susan. 1997. *Questioning Misfortune: The Pragmatics of Uncertainty in Eastern Uganda*. Cambridge: Cambridge University Press.

Richards, Audrey. 1939. *Land, Labour and Diet in Northern Rhodesia: An Economic Study of the Bemba Tribe*. London: Oxford University Press.

———. 1969 [orig. 1940]. *Bemba Marriage and Present Economic Conditions*. Livingstone: Rhodes-Livingstone Institute Paper, No. 4.

———. 1982 [orig. 1956]. *Chisungu: A Girl's Initiation Ceremony among the Bemba of Zambia*. London: Tavistock Publications.

Richter, Linda and Robert Morrell. 2006. *Baba: Men and Fatherhood in South Africa*. Cape Town: HSRC Press.

Ritchie, J. F. 1943. *The African as Suckling and Adult*. Livingstone: Rhodes-Livingstone Paper, No. 9.

Rivers, K. and P. Aggleton. 1999. *Adolescent Sexuality, Gender and the HIV Epidemic*. New York: United Nations Development Programme.

Rude, Darlene. 1999. "Reasonable Men and Provocative Women: An Analysis of Gendered Domestic Homicide in Zambia." *Journal of Southern African Studies* 25 (1): 7–27.

Sabo, Donald and David F. Gordon. 1995. *Masculinity, Health and Illness*. London: Sage.

Sanders, Todd. 1999. "'Doing Gender' in Africa." In *Those Who Play with Fire: Gender, Fertility and Transformation in East and Southern Africa*, ed. Henrietta Moore, Todd Sanders, and Bwire Kaare. 41–82. London: Athlone Press.

Santow, Gigi. 1993. "Coitus Interruptus in the 20th Century." *Population and Development Review* 19: 767–793.

Savran, David. 1998. *Taking It Like a Man*. Princeton, NJ: Princeton University Press.

Schechner, Richard. 1985. *Between Theater and Anthropology*. Philadelphia: University of Pennsylvania Press.

Schneider, Peter and Jane Schneider. 1995. "Coitus Interruptus and Family Respectability in Catholic Europe: A Sicilian Case Study." In *Conceiving the New World Order*, ed. Faye D. Ginsburg and Rayna Rapp. 177–194. Berkeley: University of California Press.

Schoepf, Brooke. 1992. "Women at Risk: Case Studies from Zaire." In *The Time of AIDS: Social Analysis, Theory and Method*, ed. Gilbert Herdt and Shirley Lindenbaum. 259–286. London: Sage Publications.

———. 1993. "AIDS Action Research with Women in Kinshasa, Zaire." *Social Science and Medicine* 37 (11): 1401–1413.

———. 1995. "Culture, Sex Research and AIDS Prevention in Africa." In *Culture and Sexual Risk: Anthropological Perspectives on AIDS*, ed. H. T. Brummelhuis and G. Herdt. 29–51. New York and Amsterdam: Gordon and Breach.

———. 2001. "International AIDS Research in Anthropology: Taking a Critical Perspective on the Crisis." *Annual Review of Anthropology* 30: 335–361.

Schuster, Ilsa M. 1979. *New Women of Lusaka*. Palo Alto, CA: Mayfield Publishing Company.

Segal, Lynne. 1990. *Slow Motion*. London: Virago.

Seidel, Gill and Rosalind Coleman. 1999. "Gender, Disclosure, Care and Decision Making in KwaZulu-Natal, South Africa: A Pilot Programme Using Storytelling Techniques." In *Families and Communities Responding to AIDS*, ed. Peter Aggleton, Graham Hart, and Peter Davies. 53–65. London: UCL Press.

Serpell, Robert. 1993. *The Significance of Schooling*. Cambridge: Cambridge University Press.

Setel, Philip W. 1999. *A Plague of Paradoxes: AIDS, Culture, and Demography in Northern Tanzania*. Chicago: University of Chicago Press.

Shire, Chenjerai. 1994. "Men Don't Go to the Moon: Language, Space and Masculinities in Zimbabwe." In *Dislocating Masculinity*, ed. Andrea Cornwall and Nancy Lindisfarne. 147–158. London: Routledge.

Silberschmidt, Margrethe. 2004. "Men, Male Sexuality and HIV/AIDS: Reflections from Studies in Rural and Urban East Africa." *Transformation* 24: 42–58.

———. 2005. "Poverty, Male Disempowerment, and Male Sexuality: Rethinking Men and Masculinities in Rural and Urban East Africa." In *African Masculinities: Men in Africa from the Late Nineteenth Century to the Present*, ed. Lahoucine Ouzgane and Robert Morrell. 189–203. London and New York: Palgrave Macmillan.

Simooya, Oscar and Nawa Sanjobo. 2001. " 'In but Free'—an HIV/AIDS Intervention in an African Prison." *Culture, Health and Sexuality* 3 (2): 241–251.

Simpson, Anthony. 2002. *The Measure of a Man*. Stockholm: Save The Children, Sweden.

———. 2003. *"Half-London" in Zambia: Contested Identities in a Catholic Mission School*. Edinburgh: Edinburgh University Press for the International African Institute.

———. 2005. "Sons and Fathers/Boys to Men in the Time of AIDS: Learning Masculinity in Zambia." *Journal of Southern African Studies* 31 (3): 569–586.

REFERENCES

Simpson, Anthony and Brian Heap. 2002. *Process Drama: A Way of Changing Attitudes*. Stockholm, Sweden: Save the Children.
Slack, Paul. 1992. "Introduction." In *Epidemics and Ideas: Essays on the Historical Perception of Pestilence*, ed. Terence Ranger and Paul Slack. 1–20. Cambridge: Cambridge University Press.
Smith, Kirsten P. and Susan Cotts Watkins. 2005. "Perceptions of Risk and Strategies for Prevention: Responses to HIV/AIDS in Rural Malawi." *Social Science and Medicine* 60: 649–660.
Sobo, Elisa. 1995. *Choosing Unsafe Sex: AIDS Risk Denial among Disadvantaged Women*. Philadelphia: University of Pennsylvania Press.
Stambach, Amy. 1998. "Too Much Studying Makes Me Crazy: School-Related Illnesses on Mount Kilimanjaro." *Comparative Education Review* 42: 497–512.
Stoler, Ann Laura. 1991. "Carnal Knowledge and Imperial Power: Gender, Race and Morality in Colonial Asia." In *Gender at the Crossroads of Knowledge: Feminist Anthropology in the Postmodern Era*, ed. M. di Leonardo. 51–101. Berkeley: University of California Press.
Takyi, B. K. 2003. "Religion and Women's Health in Ghana: Insights into HIV/AIDS Preventive and Protective Behavior." *Social Science and Medicine* 56: 1221–1234.
Tamale, Sylvia. 2001. "Think Globally, Act Locally: Using International Treaties for Women's Empowerment in East Africa." *Agenda* 50: 97–104.
Taylor, Christopher C. 1990. "Condoms and Cosmology: The 'Fractal' Person and Sexual Risk in Rwanda." *Social Science and Medicine* 31: 1023–1028.
Thomas, Felicity. 2007. "'Our Families Are Killing Us': HIV/AIDS, Witchcraft and Social Tensions in the Caprivi Region, Namibia." *Anthropology and Medicine* 14 (3): 279–291.
Thorogood, N. 1992. "Sex Education as Social Control." *Critical Public Health* 3 (4): 43–50.
Turner, Victor W. 1974. *The Ritual Process*. Harmondsworth: Penguin Books.
———. 1982. *From Ritual to Theatre: The Human Seriousness of Play*. New York: PAJ Publications.
Turner, Victor W. and Edward Bruner, ed. 1986. *The Anthropology of Experience*. Urbana, IL: University of Illinois Press.
Turshen, Meredith. 1998. "The Political Ecology of AIDS in Africa." In *The Political Economy of AIDS*, ed. Merrill Singer. 169–184. Amityville, NY: Baywood Publishing Company, Inc.
Tuzin, Donald. 1997. *The Cassowary's Revenge: The Life and Death of Masculinity in a New Guinean Society*. Chicago: Chicago University Press.
Uebel, Michael. 1997. "Men in Color." In *Race and the Subject of Masculinities*, ed. Harry Stecopoulos and Michael Uebel. Durham and London: Duke University Press.
UNAIDS. 2001. Press Release, 7 October 2001.
UNAIDS AIDS Epidemic Update 2006. Available as a pdf file at: www.unaids.org/en/HIV_data/epi2006/.

UNAIDS AIDS Epidemic Update 2007. Available as a pdf file at: www.unaids.org/en/HIV_data/epi2007/.

UNAIDS/WHO. 2004. *Epidemiological Fact Sheets on HIV/AIDS and Sexually Transmitted Infections, 2004 Update, Zambia.*

UNICEF. 2006. UNICEF Humanitarian Action Report. United Nations Children's Fund.

UNICEF. 2007. The State of the World's Children 2007. Available at: www.unicef.org/sowc07/.

Van De Wijgert, Janneke, Michael Mbizvo, Sabada Dube, Magdalene Mwale, Prisca Nyamapfeni, and Nancy Padian. 2001. "Intravaginal practises in Zimbabwe: Which Women Engage in Them or Why?" *Culture, Health and Sexuality* 3 (2): 133–148.

Vaughan, Megan. 1991. *Curing Their Ills: Colonial Power and African Illness.* Oxford: Polity Press.

———. 1992. "Syphilis in Colonial East and Central Africa: The Social Construction of an Epidemic." In *Epidemics and Ideas: Essays on the Historical Perception of Pestilence*, ed. Terence Ranger and Paul Slack. 269–302. Cambridge: Cambridge University Press.

Walker, Liz. 2005. "Men Behaving Differently: South African Men since 1994." *Culture, Health and Sexuality* 7 (3): 225–238.

Warenius, Linnéa, Karen O. Pettersson, Eva Nissen, Bengt Höjer, Petronella Chishimba, and Elizabeth Faxelid. 2007. "Vulnerability and Sexual and Reproductive Health among Zambian Secondary School Students." *Culture, Health and Sexuality* 9 (5): 533–544.

Weeks, Jeffrey. 1995. "History, Desire and Identities." In *Conceiving Sexuality: Approaches to Sex Research in a Postmodern World*, ed. Richard G. Parker and John H. Gagnon. 33–50. New York and London: Routledge.

———. 1999. "Myths and Fictions in Modern Sexualities." In *A Dangerous Knowing: Sexuality, Pedagogy and Popular Culture*, ed. Debbie Epstein and James T. Sears. 11–24. London and New York. Casssell.

Werbner, Richard P. 1991. *Tears of the Dead: The Social Biography of an African Family.* Washington, DC: Smithsonian Institution Press.

White, Luise. 1990. *The Comforts of Home; Prostitution in Colonial Nairobi.* Chicago and London: Chicago University Press.

Wilton, Tamsin and Peter Aggleton. 1991. "Condoms, Coercion and Control: Heterosexuality and the Limits to HIV/AIDS Education." In *AIDS: Responses, Interventions and Care*, ed. Peter Aggleton, Graham Hart, and Peter Davies. 149–156. London: The Falmer Press.

INDEX

abortion, 59, 68, 71, 79, 99, 100, 164, 211
abstinence, 16, 53, 54, 171, 176, 177, 178, 179, 190, 199, 217
Adam, 142, 149
and Eve, 132, 149, 151
Adams, Vincanne, 16, 140
adultery, 74, 161, 164, 211
Agadjanian, V., 216
Agatha, 105, 106, 107, 185
Aggleton, Peter, 5, 6, 214, 218
Ahlberg, Beth M., 208, 212
AIDS
  biomedical explanations for, 7, 154, 156, 169, 170, 191
  conspiracy to kill Africans, 155
  deaths of family and friends, 155, 156, 157, 165, 169, 171, 190, 208
  empathy, 200
  HIV/AIDS competence, 196
  liberatory potential of, 8, 203
  prevention campaigns, 7, 16, 171–3, 176, 189, 190–1, 200
  and religion, 5, 145, 156, 216
  shame, 145
Akeroyd, Anne V., 206
alcohol
  influence of, 50, 96, 102, 114, 139, 175–6, 190
Anne, 110–12
antiretroviral therapy (ART), 16, 166, 171, 172, 190, 194
aphrodisiacs, 44, 117, 118

banacimbusa (women marriage instructors), 82, 83, 84, 86, 114, 119, 141
Barnett, Tony, 217, 219
Bawa Yamba, C., 156
Bayley, Anne, 2
Baylies, Carolyn, 6, 10, 202, 203, 206
beer, *see* alcohol
Bible, 15, 54, 55, 73, 89, 126, 128, 132, 143, 199
Boal, Augusto, 218
Bolton, Ralph, 10
Bond, V. A., 59
Bowell, Pamela, 196
Bruner, Jerome, 195, 196
Bujra, Janet, 6, 10, 202, 203, 206, 210
Butler, Judith, 9, 193, 196, 203

Caldwell, J. C., 212, 213
Caldwell, P., 212, 213
Campbell, Carole A., 6
Campbell, Catherine, 206
Catherine, 76
Catholics, 4, 15, 53, 56, 148, 165, 217
celibacy, 55, 177
Chalwe, 110, 111, 112
Chege, Fatuma, 207
Chileshe, 166, 168
Chimbala, 51, 63, 64, 145–6
chisungu, see cisungu
Christianity, 15, 16, 85, 113, 149, 155
  Born Again, 15, 161, 167, 169, 189

Christianity—*continued*
  Christian identity, 3, 73
  church membership, 4, 145, 164
  conversion, 15, 161, 165, 166, 169
  religious education, 52–3
Christopher, 37
circumlocution, 159, 216
cisungu, 82, 210
coitus interruptus (withdrawal), *see* sex
colonialism, 5, 203
Colson, Elizabeth, 21, 22, 29, 85, 91, 148, 149, 164, 169, 202, 206, 207, 208, 210, 211, 213, 215
compassion, 34, 157, 159, 169, 200
condoms
  association with promiscuity, 84, 145, 171, 179
  association with prostitution, 50, 175
  barrier to intimacy, 140, 190
  bursts during intercourse, 96, 102, 122, 139
  Catholic Church opposition to, 4, 161, 176, 177
  efficacy doubted, 91, 190
  female condoms, 141
  and Kenneth Kaunda, 173
  non-availability in prisons, 134
  promotion opposed, 16, 171, 189
  and reduction of pleasure, 141
  and religious education, 53
condom use
  and alcohol, 139
  and "class" of sexual partner, 51, 52, 59, 95
  and faith in girls, 49, 50
  at first intercourse, 48, 125
  estimates of condom use, 59
  at university, 71
Connell, Robert, 5, 6, 8, 9, 42, 195, 196, 201, 206, 218
contraception, 84, 142, 176, 215, 217
  pill, 50, 84, 142, 176, 214

cross-border trade, 67, 69, 107
cross-cousins
  first teachers in sex, 43
  marriage between, 207–8

dagga (marijuana), 50
Darius
  on cleaning after sex, 87, 88
  on condoms, 50
  on European sex, 115–16
  fear of AIDS, 73
  on HIV test, 180
  on homosexuality, 134
  on masturbation, 126
  on oral sex, 129
  on premature ejaculation, 137
  sex in childhood and adolescence, 37, 42, 46
  sexual abuse, 40
  on sexual control, 136
  on tight and dry sex, 120
  on wife-beating, 27
David
  on extra-marital affair, 183
  fear of witchcraft, 154
  on HIV test, 183–4
  reconversion, 165
  sex in childhood, 42
Demba, 3, 153
denial, 114, 185, 212
depression, 4, 77, 82, 146, 156, 159, 181, 186, 191
Devil, *see* Satan
discipline
  father's discipline, 13, 25–30, 34
divorce, 21, 32, 80, 96, 99, 107, 114, 212, 217
Dominic
  on cleaning after sex, 87
  on first sex, 45
  on homosexuality, 132–3
  on masturbation, 55
  on *muti*, 44
  on peer pressure at university, 70
  on self-control, 136
Doreen, 102

Dover, Paul, 34, 39, 45, 54, 59, 207, 208, 209, 211, 214
Dowsett, Gary, 7

Edmund
  on "African sexuality," 116
  on condoms, 51–2, 71, 208
  on relationship with father, 31–2
  on self-control, 137
Edward, 81
Eileen, 177, 178, 184
Elizabeth, 145–6, 161, 178, 215
Enoch
  awareness of sex, 38
  on brother's death, 160
  first sex, 40–1
  on HIV test, 182
  marriage of, 77
  on masturbation, 55
  on *muti*, 44, 182
  pregnancy of girlfriend, 53–4
  on tight and dry sex, 120
Epstein, Arnold L., 92, 113, 206, 211
Esau, 157–8
ethnographic fieldwork, 3
evolution, 15, 149

Fanon, Frantz, 10
Farmer, Paul, 206
father-son relationship, 13, 20, 31, 32, 34, 52
  discipline, 13, 25–30, 34
fears
  of appearing weak, 138
  of HIV, 13, 179, 190, 192
  of mystical harm, 86
  of pregnancies, 65
  of venereal disease, 65
  of witchcraft, 157
  wives' fears, 15, 114, 170, 180, 184
Feldman, Douglas, 58
Ferguson, James, 92, 114, 213
fertility
  core of manhood, 59
  importance for Goba, 45, 59
  women's fertility, 76

first-born, 20, 101, 206
Flood, Michael, 59
Foucault, M, 10
frame
  frame analysis, 196
  in process drama, 197, 200
Frankenberg, Ronald, 156
Freire, Paolo, 196
funerals, 171

Garner, Robert C., 156
gender
  gender-appropriate tasks, 22–3
  gender identities, 5, 201
  gender ideologies, 6
  gender inequality, 206
  gender propriety, 136
  and *lobola*, 74
  performance of, 196
  in process drama, 197–200
gender relations
  ambiguities in, 202
  in colonial period, 91–2
  mutability in, 203
Genesis, Book of, 15, 49, 142, 149, 151, 209
George
  on homosexuality, 133–4
  on masturbation, 126
  on oral sex, 128–9
  on satisfying wife, 123
  on self-control, 136
  on tight and dry sex, 121
  on withdrawal, 124–5
Goba, 39, 45, 207, 208, 211, 214
God
  AIDS, punishment from God, 160–4
  belief in, 15, 49, 145, 148
  faith in God to cure AIDS, 16, 170, 184, 190
  gender of, 149
  giver of children, 79, 106, 208
  Leza/Lesa, 148, 149, 169, 230
  and prosperity, 166
  teenage ideas of, 147–52

Goffman, Erving, 195, 196, 197
gonorrhea, 49, 69, 180
Grace, 74, 87
grieving, 217
Gutmann, Matthew, 206

Hall, Stuart, 9
Hambayi
 childhood sex, 40
 on condoms, 50
 death of first wife, 33
 first marriage of, 78
 on God, 151-2
 on homosexuality, 133
 on masturbation, 55
 mentors of, 24, 41
 relationship with father, 23
 second marriage of, 105-7
 on self-control, 137
Hansen, Karen, 92, 93, 113, 212
Harold, 27
Heald, Suzette, 7, 8, 87, 212
Heap, Brian, 195, 196, 218
Henry
 on celibacy, 177
 on condoms, 178-9
 divorce of, 211
 on double standards, 49
 first sexual intercourse, 43
 on future wife, 65
 on God, 150, 151-2, 162
 on HIV test, 184
 on homosexuality, 133
 marriage of, 73, 75, 107-9
 on primary boarding school, 30
 on shaving, 89
Hinfelaar, Hugo, 55, 148, 149, 164, 215
HIV
 suspicions of HIV status, 166, 172, 183
HIV risk, 60, 70, 91, 94, 114, 145, 173-6, 190, 194
HIV test, 16, 172, 179-85, 189, 190-1, 194, 195

homosexuality, 39, 55, 56, 128, 130-4, 140, 143, 214
household budgets, 97, 110, 112
Hunter, Mark, 48

Iliffe, John, 2, 172, 205, 216
incest, 207
infidelity
 "African infidelity," 134-5
 mystical dangers of, 138
 suspicions of, 33, 88, 89, 92, 102, 107, 108, 118, 165
initiation
 student initiation, 54
 of women, 121, 202, 207, 212, 218
interviews
 language of, 12

jealousy, 15, 153-4
Jeater, Diana, 85, 155, 209
Jesus, 148, 161
Josephine, 99-100
Joshua, 33
 marriage of, 93-4, 113
Justina, 104

Kabwe, 64, 145
Kalulu, 172
Kangwa, 1, 23
 on ART, 194
 childhood sex, 38
 on condoms, 49
 on exchange in sex, 48
 on future wife, 63-4
 on God, 161-2
 on HIV test, 181-2
 on homosexuality, 130
 illness, 149-50
 marriage, 76
 on wife-beating, 25-6
Kaposi's sarcoma, 2, 139, 166
Kaufman, Michael, 9, 218
Kaunda, Kenneth, 173, 217
Kimmel, Michael, 9

Index

kissing, 116, 208, 213
kitchen parties, 109, 212

labia
   stretching of, 119, 208, 213
labor migration, 91
Laqueur, Thomas, 209
Last, Murray, 206
Leonard, 32, 42
life histories, 10–12
Lillian, 101–2
Lizzie, 99
lobola (bridewealth), 14, 74–5, 79, 81, 90, 210
Lonsdale, John, 155
love, 51, 63, 65, 101, 114, 126, 135, 142
   beating as sign of, 84
   love potions, 44, 62, 211
Lupton, Deborah, 7

Mabvuto, 74, 87, 88
Malama, 68
   on "African sexuality," 116
   on anal sex, 127
   on aphrodisiacs, 118
   marriage of, 77, 88
   on withdrawal, 124
manhood, 9, 19, 23, 25, 45, 46, 51, 54, 57, 59
manliness, 5, 8, 35, 194, 195
mantomba (children's game), 22
Margaret (Sampa's mother), 39, 74, 164, 176, 210
marijuana (*dagga*), 50
Marks, Shula, 10
marriage, 4, 15, 60, 169, 202
   absence of communication in, 15, 91, 123, 181, 185, 191
   Bemba marriage pot, 90, 210
   companionship, 63, 91, 110
   cross-cousin marriage, 207–8
   customary marriage, 74
   distrust in, 65, 92, 93, 114

"English manners," 93
   ideal age for marriage, 14
   importance of children, 79–82
   marriage instruction, 14, 82–6, 89, 90, 104, 109, 112, 119, 210
   married life, 91–114
   roles of husband and wife, 97, 106, 108
Martha, 168, 184
masculinities, 5–10
   instability of, 48
   range of, 113, 201
masculinity
   fragility of, 9, 201
   ideologies of, 7, 17, 194
   performance of, 7, 8, 201
   and pretence, 49, 141, 202, 203
masturbation
   in adolescence, 55–8
   in adulthood, 125–7
   association with homosexuality, 130
   mutual masturbation, 133, 142, 208–9
   sin of Onan, 209
Matilda, 76, 77, 94
Maxwell, 66–7
Mbilinyi, Majorie, 11
memory, 10, 19, 35, 37, 206
men
   "breadwinners," 14, 61, 108, 113, 203
   and emotion, 47
   and force, 14, 25, 42, 66
   hunting for women, 91, 141
   independence, 30, 65, 113
   patriarchal dividend, 194
   "real men," 7, 19, 25, 47, 48, 55, 79, 94, 113, 124, 213
   and strength, 25, 39, 44, 57, 58, 116, 123, 137, 141, 190
   superiority claims of, 16, 25, 87, 136, 149
   vulnerability of men, 5

menstruation, 50, 80, 99, 108, 109, 127, 210
  menstrual blood, 84
  sexual intercourse during, 58, 127, 129
mentors, 24, 41, 47
Miescher, Stephan, 8, 206
misogyny, 92, 114
missionaries, 55, 56, 60, 133, 148, 150, 169, 217
  Catholic Brothers, 54
modernity, 94, 119, 128, 140
Mogensen, H. O., 164
money
  excitement of, 190
Moore, Henrietta, 91
Morrell, Robert, 6, 143, 207
mother-son relationship, 13, 21, 92, 191
"movious," 77, 147, 174
Mugabe, Robert, 143
Mulenga, 78, 79
  infertility of, 80–1
Mutale, 75, 146, 179
  on marriage, 109–11
muti, 44, 58, 84, 86, 94, 99, 117, 213
Mutinta
  on Catholic marriage instruction, 73–4
  depression, 146
  on father, 22
  on future wife, 64
  on God, 151
  on homosexuality, 130
  on *lobola*, 74–5, 79
  on marriage, 109–10
  on prevention campaigns, 179
  at university, 70–1
Mwanakatwe, John, 53
Mwanza, 102, 138, 139

Ndubani, Phillimon, 41, 46, 139, 211, 213
Niehaus, Isaak, 207
nightmares of students, 152, 194

nsalamu, 74, 210
Nujoma, Sam, 143

Obbo, Caroline, 6, 218
Okely, Judith, 5

Pamela
  divorce, 211
  on God, 162
  on *lobola*, 75
  marriage, 107–9
  on prevention campaigns, 179, 184
  on shaving, 89
Parikh, Shanti A., 210, 213
Parker, Richard G., 3, 5, 7, 10, 206, 214, 218
Pattman, Rob, 130, 207
Paul, 1, 47, 71–2, 193
  on Catholic priests, 177
  on deaths of siblings, 165–8
  on future wife, 65
  on hell, 148
  on homosexuality, 132
  marriage of, 76–7
  on masturbation, 56
  relationship with father, 20, 24, 25, 26, 27–8, 33
  on stepmother, 21
  on trust in marriage, 94–5
peer pressure, 14, 46, 59, 70, 76, 90
penis
  cleaning after sex, 86–8
  handling of, 127
  size of, 44, 56
  symbol of power, 9
Pentecostals, 85, 86, 149, 156, 161, 165, 166, 168, 169, 184
PEPFAR (American President's Fund), 190, 217
Peter, 193
  on cleaning after sex, 88
  delayed first intercourse, 66
  on fighting, 24
  on HIV test, 172, 194
  on masturbation, 55

relationship with father, 30–1
on shaving, 89
Pigg, Stacey Leigh, 16, 140
Piot, Peter, 6
Plummer, Ken, 6, 11
polygamy, 62, 81, 161
Powdermaker, Hortense, 92, 206
precedence, 149, 215
pregnancies, 39, 53, 65, 53, 75–8
process drama, 16, 195–201
Promise, 1, 12
on "African infidelity," 135
on anal sex, 128, 214
on cleaning after sex, 87
death of, 195
depression, 156
on Esau's death, 156–8, 163
first penetrative intercourse, 43–4
on HIV risk, 173–5
on HIV test, 180
on homosexuality, 130–1
"loose," 66
marriage of, 77–8, 82–3, 100–5
on masturbation, 57–8, 126
on polygamy, 62
relationship with father, 28–9
schoolgirl pregnancy, 54
on self-control, 138
on styles of sex, 122–3

Ranger, Terence, 155
Rasing, Thera, 207, 208, 210
Rebecca, 78, 105
Reid, Elizabeth, 5, 200
religious ideas, 143, 147–52
  afterlife, 15, 148, 150, 151, 152
respect, 20, 31, 34, 38, 74, 86, 96, 119, 141, 172, 197
  bulemu (Tonga), 20
Reynaud, E., 9
Reynolds-Whyte, Susan, 154
Richards, Audrey, 21, 38, 54, 85, 90, 91, 164, 193, 202, 203, 206, 207, 208, 210, 211, 212, 213, 214, 215, 216, 217

risk
  to manliness, 7
  of pregnancies, 49, 50
Robert, 71–2, 143, 166–8
Rude, Darlene, 92
Ruth, 80–1, 95, 96–8, 129, 186

Sampa, 1
  on "African infidelity", 134–5
  on AIDS stigma, 159–60
  on aphrodisiacs, 118
  on beer, 139
  on childhood sex, 43
  on cleaning after sex, 87
  on condoms, 49–50, 68–9, 178
  on "dancing in bed," 121–2
  first marriage, 78–9
  on God, 150, 163
  on homosexuality, 133
  illness, 185–9
  on masturbation, 127
  relationship with father, 33
  on risks, 175–6
  second marriage, 80–1, 95–100
  on self-control, 137–8
  on sexual abuse, 39–40
  on shaving, 88–9
  on tight and dry sex, 120
  on witchcraft, 156
  on withdrawal, 125
Sanders, Todd, 6
Sarah, 94
Satan, 150, 163, 176
Savran, David, 201
Schechner, Richard, 196
Schoepf, Brooke, 4, 206, 216, 218
Schuster, Ilsa M., 92
Segal, Lynne, 208
semen
  and condoms, 140–1
  consistency of, 45
  as dirt, 90
  proper place of semen, 122, 142
  wasting semen, 55, 129, 214
Serpell, Robert, 209

Setel, Philip W., 6, 10, 177, 215, 216, 219
Seventh Day Adventists, 4, 24, 55, 126, 151, 166, 168, 178, 215
sex
  anal sex, 127, 128, 132, 214
  "carelessness" in sex, 49, 52, 76, 162, 168, 172, 191
  ejaculation, 8, 41, 44, 50, 55 56, 57, 59, 84, 96, 119, 120, 122, 125, 127, 137
  exchange in sex, 40, 48, 68, 86, 89, 95, 131, 212
  excitement in sex, 41, 68
  extramarital sex, 15, 48, 91, 93, 114, 118, 122, 161, 169, 216
  groups in first sex, 40
  hydaulic model of, 15, 141
  intergenerational communication about, 197, 207
  learning sex in childhood games, 22, 37, 38
  "loose", 66, 67, 76, 89, 102, 115
  missionary position, 207
  oral sex, 97, 107, 128–30, 141, 214
  penetration, 8, 38, 41, 116, 126, 127, 129, 130
  premarital sex, 14, 45, 54, 58–9, 85, 90, 149, 156, 161
  respectability in sex, 122, 136, 190
  rounds of sex, 14, 45, 123–4, 141, 214
  "safe period," 51
  sex with parallel cousins, 43
  sex with schoolgirls, 53, 67, 69, 78, 81, 89, 208
  styles, 122, 193
  tight and dry sex, 45, 118–21, 191, 213
  unprotected sex, 60, 70, 71, 72, 89, 95, 96, 102, 173, 190
  violent imagery of, 14
  "wet dreams," 39, 137
  "wet sex," 116, 213
  withdrawal, 124, 125, 209, 214
sexual abuse, 39, 60
sexual competence, 58, 124, 193
sexual conquest, 8, 35, 41, 58, 119, 141, 194, 201
sexual control, 137
sexual debut, *see* sexual intercourse
sexual intercourse
  first sexual intercourse, 24, 41, 46, 47, 48, 193, 207
sexual performance, 9, 55, 117
sexuality, 5, 8, 9, 10, 155, 196
  "African sexuality," 15, 93, 140, 212, 213
  "European sexuality," 115, 116
shaving of pubic hair, 88–90
Shire, Chenjerai, 206
Silberschmidt, Margrethe, 6, 9
silence
  African gift of, 39, 132
Simon
  on double standards, 93
  on female sexuality, 121
  on God, 163
  on HIV test, 172, 181
  on homosexuality, 133
  illness, 185
  on masturbation, 126
  pressure to marry, 82
  relationship with father, 31
  on university, 70
sin
  Kenneth Kaunda, 173
  and premarital sex, 45, 54, 59, 68, 149
  and sexual shame, 155, 156
Slack, Paul, 155
sport, 42, 70
Stella, 88, 159, 173, 180
stepmothers, 21, 24, 62
stigma, 145, 147, 159, 172, 190, 199
Susan, 77–8, 100–4
Swart, Sandra, 6, 143
syphilis, 69, 140

Index

TB, 129, 137, 146, 147, 157, 160, 166, 181, 182, 185, 186, 187, 188, 189, 194
teachers
  AIDS deaths of, 209
  corporal punishment, 30
  sexual exploitation of schoolgirls, 43, 46, 66
tradition, 15, 62, 74, 75, 79, 83, 85, 86, 87, 88, 89, 90, 96, 119, 128, 140, 181, 190
traditional medicine, *see muti*
trust
  absence of trust between husbands and wives, 13, 15, 93, 102, 104, 107, 109, 184, 185, 191
  between mothers and sons, 92
  and rejection of condoms, 50, 59, 71
Turner, Victor W., 195, 196, 197
Turshen, Meredith, 205
Tuzin, Donald, 9

ukondoloka (to grow thin), 164
umucinshi (respect), 20
UNAIDS, 2, 6, 155, 205
uncertainty, 154, 155, 159, 169, 172, 185, 188, 191
UNICEF, 3, 241
UNIP (United National Independence Party), 1, 53
university, 69–72, 110, 111, 146

Vaughan, Megan, 91, 140, 155, 213
venereal disease, 52
  bolabola, 69

village
  reference point for "African sexuality," 116
  synonym for tradition, 128
violence
  as affirmation of manhood, 23
  in compounds, 97
  of fathers toward sons, 25, 28, 29, 31, 207
  of men toward women, 27, 35, 92
Virgin Birth, 148
virginity, 85
virility, 14, 202
Voluntary Counseling and Testing (VCT), 16, 171, 194

Walker, Liz, 206
weddings, 74, 75, 86, 108, 110, 111
Weeks, Jeffrey, 9, 219
Werbner, Richard, 206
White, Luise, 217
Whiteside, Alan, 217
Wilton, Tamsin, 5
witchcraft, 16, 33, 50, 87, 131, 140, 152–8, 159, 207, 215
  student nightmares, 152, 194
women
  violence toward, 5, 35, 41, 84, 108, 146, 202, 206, 207
  wives as men's teachers in sex, 86, 129

Zambia Demographic and Health Survey 2001–2002, 35, 207, 214

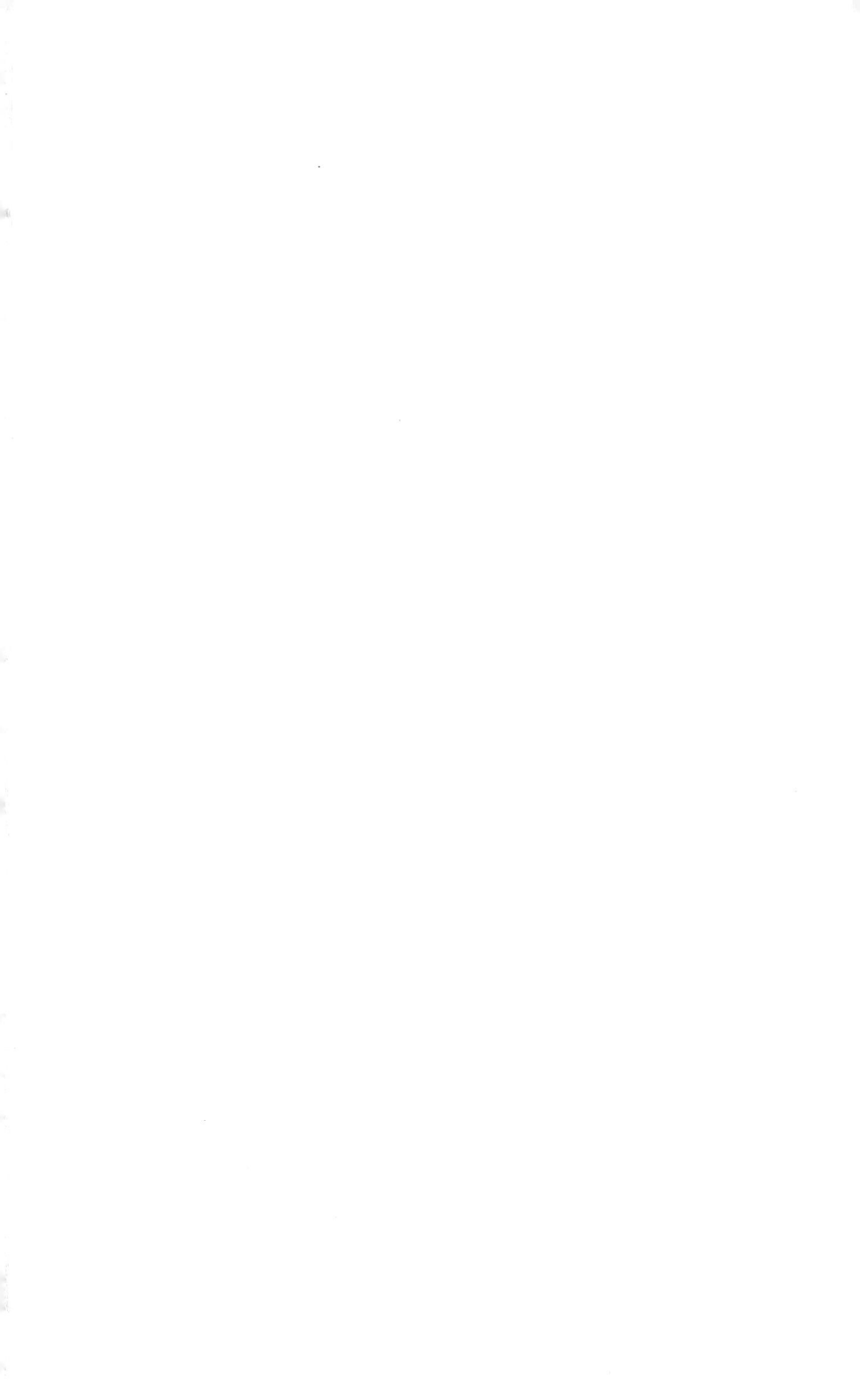